Neuromuscular Disease:
A Case-Based Approach

Neuromuscular Disease: A Case-Based Approach

John H. J. Wokke
Professor of Neurology, Department of Neurology and Neurosurgery, Rudolf Magnus Institute of Neuroscience,
University Medical Center Utrecht, the Netherlands

Pieter A. van Doorn
Professor of Neuromuscular Disorders, Department of Neurology, Erasmus MC, University Medical Center Rotterdam, the Netherlands

Jessica E. Hoogendijk
Neurologist, Department of Neurology, Rudolf Magnus Institute of Neuroscience, University Medical Center Utrecht, the Netherlands

Marianne de Visser
Professor of Neuromuscular Disorders, Department of Neurology, Academic Medical Center Amsterdam, the Netherlands

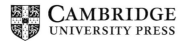

CAMBRIDGE
UNIVERSITY PRESS

CAMBRIDGE
UNIVERSITY PRESS

University Printing House, Cambridge CB2 8BS, United Kingdom

Cambridge University Press is part of the University of Cambridge.

It furthers the University's mission by disseminating knowledge in the pursuit of
education, learning and research at the highest international levels of excellence.

www.cambridge.org
Information on this title: www.cambridge.org/9780521171854

First published 2013
Reprinted 2017

Printed in the United Kingdom by Clays, St Ives plc.

A catalogue record for this publication is available from the British Library

Library of Congress Cataloguing in Publication data
Neuromuscular disease : a case-based approach / John H. J. Wokke . . . [et al.].
    p.   ;   cm.
Includes bibliographical references and index.
ISBN 978-0-521-17185-4 (pbk.)
I. Wokke, John H. J., 1952–
[DNLM: 1. Neuromuscular Diseases – diagnosis – Case Reports.   2. Neuromuscular Diseases – therapy – Case
Reports.   3. Diagnosis, Differential – Case Reports. WE 550]
616.8–dc23

                                                                              2012035669

ISBN 978-0-521-17185-4 Paperback

Additional resources for this publication at www.cambridge.org/9780521171854

Contents

Section 4 Myopathies

Preface

Neuromuscular diseases are a fascinating aspect of neurology. Careful history taking and dedicated neurological examination generally enable the clinician to localize the disease within the nervous or muscular system, and to make a clinical and differential diagnosis. Measuring blood values, such as glucose level and creatine kinase activity, and other easily accessible ancillary tests, like electromyography, nerve conduction studies, and imaging tools, help to refine that diagnosis.

In many patients with a suspected neuromuscular disorder, the next steps may include advanced analysis of skeletal muscle biopsies, using immunohistochemistry and Western blots to characterize a wide range of proteins, and a rapidly expanding number of genetic tests. There has been a spectacular advance in knowledge of hereditary neuromuscular diseases over the past decade. The discovery of manifold genes and mutations has led to a considerable broadening of phenotypes that form a new challenge for the clinician.

Generally speaking, the diagnostic process is rewarding, as patients want to hear what the diagnosis is. Usually, a diagnosis comes as a relief. Once the diagnosis has been made, patients and their families can be informed about prognosis, presence of hereditary aspects, and treatment that can be given. Treatment options include immunosuppression, immunomodulation, or a combination in a wide spectrum of immune-mediated neuromuscular diseases ranging from a progressive disease such as Guillain–Barré syndrome (GBS) to a more chronic disease like classic myasthenia gravis. Pompe disease is the first hereditary metabolic neuromuscular disease in which it was found that enzyme replacement therapy can induce improved function. Trials with exon-skipping treatment in Duchenne muscular dystrophy have been introduced into the clinic. The effects of noninvasive respiratory support and devices that help to preserve function and quality of life cannot be underestimated. Most treatments are effective only if given at an early stage. This is especially true if the onset is acute.

It has been calculated that about 1% of the population suffers from a neuromuscular disease, but on the whole, individual diseases are rare. Many neuromuscular patients have to live with the consequences for the rest of their lives. In 2010, the costs of direct healthcare, direct nonmedical support, and indirect costs due to neuromuscular diseases, irrespective of who was footing the bill, were estimated to amount to 7.7 billion euro in 30 European countries, equivalent to about 1% of the total costs for all neurological and mental disorders.[1] Patients are, therefore, entitled to a timely diagnosis and treatment advice, so that society can still provide the means.

During medical training, most doctors will learn little about these rare, but characteristic and incapacitating diseases, and will not recognize the manifestations. An exceptional example is an experienced general practitioner (GP) who observed an elderly woman from his practice cycling with a dropped head. On examination, he noted only a drooping eyelid. When she complained of intermittent diplopia, he correctly suggested a diagnosis of classic myasthenia gravis. In contrast, GBS will be easily recognized by most GPs. At the other end of the spectrum, chronic diabetic neuropathy is very common and can be diagnosed easily. Even neurologists may find the diagnostic process of a neuromuscular disease cumbersome.

We, therefore, decided to write a pragmatic and accessible clinical guide, not opting for completeness or for a comprehensive textbook of which many excellent examples exist.

In this book we focus upon adult patients with a neuromuscular disease. In addition, we present some cases of patients with an alternative diagnosis that could mimic an acute or chronic neuromuscular disorder. We do not present cases of children with a neuromuscular disease albeit that some of our patients had initial complaints in late adolescence.

---

[1] Olesen J, Gustavsson A, Svensson M, et al. The economic costs of brain disorders in Europe. *Eur J Neurol* 2012; **19**: 155–162.

First, we present an overview of symptoms, signs, characteristic features, and common phenotypes. Next, we present 59 examples of neuromuscular diseases. We start with the case histories of patients from our practices. We discuss early signs, ancillary investigations, diagnosis, and disease course and treatment strategies. In the section *General remarks*, we present a brief summary of current knowledge about the cause and treatment of diseases, and about epidemiological data. The many tables are a way of clarifying what we judge to be most important in a particular topic. References are selected with emphasis on reviews or landmark papers. Where necessary, we refer to practice parameters, guidelines, and informative websites.

We realize that the field of molecular genetic diagnosis of neuromuscular disorders is moving rapidly. New genes and mutations are continuously being discovered and functions of genes and proteins unravelled. Where possible, we present the current data and try to explain mechanisms of disease. The reader is advised to check with websites for the most recent data.

Our fellow neurologists Professor Leonard van den Berg and Drs. Wim Linssen, Nicolette Notermans, Willem Oerlemans, W. Ludo van der Pol, Jan Veldink, and Alexander Vrancken commented upon individual cases. Our eminent clinical neurophysiologist Dr. Hessel Franssen commented upon the presentation of electrophysiological data and supplied the figures on needle electromyography in Case 4 and the decremental response in the classic myasthenia gravis case. Professor Baziel van Engelen and Dr. Nens van Alfen helped with the case of the patient with idiopathic neuralgic amyotrophy, and Dr. Leo Visser with the intensive care neuropathy case. Professor Jan Verschuuren helped with the anti-MuSK myasthenia gravis and the Lambert–Eaton myasthenic syndrome cases. The residents Annette Compter and Esther Verstraete helped with the figures of the patients with Lyme radiculoneuritis and amyotrophic lateral sclerosis and frontotemporal dementia, respectively, and Christiaan Saris filmed the Babinski and Chaddock signs. Professor Jan van Gijn kindly provided the figures of the patient with a neurogenic thoracic outlet syndrome. Dr. Wim Spliet, neuropathologist, provided some fine illustrative figures of muscle biopsies. Dr. Anneke van der Kooi, neurologist, and an enthusiastic reading group consisting of residents, Sefanja Achterberg, Aysun Altinbas, Marieke van Oijen, Stephan Wens, and Beatrijs Wokke, furnished invaluable comments that kept our feet on the ground. We are extremely grateful to them all.

Most importantly, we thank our patients, some of whom we have known for over 20 years, who form the basis of this book. They have helped us to expand our knowledge. We also thank them for their willingness to help with the illustrations. One photograph or video can teach clinicians more than pages of text. We hope our selection of illustrating cases of patients with neuromuscular diseases will motivate our readers to join us in a tour through this part of the fascinating field of neurology, the neuromuscular diseases.

December 2012
Utrecht, Rotterdam, and Amsterdam, the Netherlands
John Wokke
Pieter van Doorn
Jessica Hoogendijk
Marianne de Visser

Abbreviations

ACE	angiotensin-converting enzyme	EMG	needle electromyography
AChR	acetylcholine receptor	ERT	enzyme-replacement therapy
A-CIDP	acute-onset chronic inflammatory demyelinating polyneuropathy	ESR	erythrocyte sedimentation rate
		FALS	familial ALS
AD	autosomal dominant	FDG-PET	fluorodeoxyglucose–positron emission tomography
AIDP	acute inflammatory demyelinating polyneuropathy		
		FSHD	facioscapulohumeral dystrophy
ALS	amyotrophic lateral sclerosis	FTD	frontotemporal dementia
AMAN	acute motor axonal neuropathy	GAA	acid alpha-glucosidase
AMSAN	acute motor and sensory axonal neuropathy	GBS	Guillain–Barré syndrome
		GSD	glycogen storage disease
AR	autosomal recessive	GP	general practitioner
BMD	Becker muscular dystrophy	HE	hematoxylin and eosin
CB	conduction block	HIV	human immunodeficiency virus
CIAP	chronic idiopathic axonal polyneuropathy	HNA	hereditary neuralgic amyotrophy
		HNPP	hereditary neuropathy with liability to pressure palsies
CIDP	chronic inflammatory demyelinating polyneuropathy		
		HPA	hypothalamus–pituitary–adrenal (axis)
CIM	critical illness myopathy	HSAN	hereditary sensory and autonomic neuropathy
CIP	critical illness polyneuropathy		
CK	creatine kinase	HSMN	hereditary sensory and motor neuropathy
CMAP	compound muscle action potential		
CMT	Charcot–Marie–Tooth	HSP	hereditary spastic paraplegia
CMV	cytomegalovirus	HTLV	human T-cell lymphocytotropic virus
CNS	central nervous system	IBM	inclusion body myositis
CPEO	chronic progressive external ophthalmoplegia	ICU	intensive care unit
		IENF	intraepidermal nerve fiber
CRP	C-reactive protein	INA	idiopathic neuralgic amyotrophy
CSF	cerebrospinal fluid	IVIg	intravenous immunoglobulins
CT	computed tomography	KSS	Kearns–Sayre syndrome
DM	myotonic dystrophy	LEMS	Lambert–Eaton myasthenic syndrome
DMD	Duchenne muscular dystrophy	LGMD	limb girdle muscular dystrophy
DML	distal motor latency	LMN	lower motor neuron
DRG	dorsal root ganglion	LOS	lipo-oligosaccharides
DSP	distal symmetric polyneuropathy	MADSAM	multifocal acquired demyelinating sensory and motor (neuropathy)
EBV	Epstein-Barr virus		
EDS	excessive day-time sleepiness	MAG	myelin-associated glycoprotein
EGRIS	Erasmus GBS Respiratory Insufficiency Scale	mEGOS	modified Erasmus GBS Outcome Scale
		MERRF	myoclonus epilepsy with ragged red fibers
ELIZA	enzyme linked immunosorbent assay		
EM	erythema migrans	MFN2	mitofusin 2

MFS	Miller–Fisher syndrome	POEMS	polyneuropathy, organomegaly, endocrinopathy, M-protein, and skin changes
MGUS	monoclonal gammopathy of undetermined significance		
MMN	multifocal motor neuropathy	POLG	polymerase gamma
MMSE	Mini-Mental State Examination	PPS	postpoliomyelitis syndrome
MMT	manual muscle testing	PROMM	proximal myotonic myopathy, myotonic dystrophic type 2
MNCV	motor nerve conduction velocity		
MND	motor neuron disease	PSMA	progressive spinal muscular atrophy
MNGIE	mitochondrial neurogastrointestinal encephalomyopathy	RCT	randomized controlled trial
		SALS	sporadic amyotrophic lateral sclerosis
MPZ	myelin protein zero	SANDO	sensory ataxic neuropathy with dysarthria and ophthalmoparesis
M-protein	monoclonal protein		
MRC	Medical Research Council	SCA	spinocerebellar ataxia
MRI	magnetic resonance imaging	SCLC	small-cell lung cancer
MS	multiple sclerosis	SDAVF	spinal dural arteriovenous fistula
MUP	motor unit potential	SFN	small fiber neuropathy
MuSK	muscle-specific kinase	sIBM	sporadic inclusion body myositis
NARP	Neuropathy, ataxia, and retinitis pigmentosa	SMA	spinal muscular atrophy
		SMN	survival motor neuron (gene)
NINDS	National Institute of Neurological Disorders and Stroke	SNAP	sensory nerve action potential
		SSRI	selective serotonin reuptake inhibitor
NIV	noninvasive ventilation	TRF	treatment-related fluctuations
NMJ	neuromuscular junction	TSH	thyroid stimulating hormone
NSAID	nonsteroidal anti-inflammatory drug	ULN	upper limit of normal
OPMD	oculopharyngeal muscular dystrophy	UMN	upper motor neuron
PCR	polymerase chain reaction	VC	vital capacity
PE	plasma exchange	VEGF	vascular endothelial growth factor
PEG	percutaneous endoscopic gastrostomy	VEP	visual evoked potential
PLS	primary lateral sclerosis	VGCC	voltage-gated calcium channel
PMA	progressive muscular atrophy	VGKC	voltage-gated potassium channel
PMP22	peripheral myelin protein 22	WNV	West Nile virus

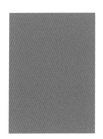

Introduction: approach to the patient

Introduction

Clinical features, rate of progression, and functional impairment of neuromuscular diseases vary between patients and diseases, even in diseases and within families with the same genetic cause. Acquired neuromuscular disease may also show great variability of symptoms and signs, progression, and response to treatment.

Yet, with a keen clinical eye and sound clinical reasoning, it is possible to establish a clinical and differential diagnosis, and to select relevant ancillary tests. In each following section, we discuss common symptoms and signs.

Time course at onset (Table 1)

"Acute" in neuromuscular disorders reflects a nadir within four weeks after onset. Initial symptoms may be in the remote past. Most hereditary diseases first manifest in childhood or adolescence, but onset at an advanced age is no exception. It is useful to ask when motor milestones were reached and whether the patient could keep up with peers at sports. A common finding in clinical neurology is that many patients with chronic disease will – due to memory activation – on returning from the first visit, recall an earlier onset of manifestations.

Table 1. Time course of neuromuscular diseases

• Acute	Nadir within 4 wk after onset
• Subacute	Progressive course lasting a maximum of 8 wk
• Chronic progressive	Progression continuing after 8 wk
• Monophasic	One single disease period
• Relapsing and remitting	Periods of worsening and improvement

Symptoms and signs of the motor system

Fatigue

Fatigue is a common initial complaint of patients with a neuromuscular disease. Examples are amyotrophic lateral sclerosis (ALS), Pompe disease, and myotonic dystrophy (DM). Fatigue may be a late or residual symptom as in patients with postpoliomyelitis syndrome, Guillain–Barré syndrome (GBS), and myositis. If fatigue is the predominant feature, without objective signs such as weakness or elevated serum creatine kinase (CK) activity, it is unlikely to be a neuromuscular disease. Chronic fatigue syndrome is not a neuromuscular disease.

Cramps

Cramps – spontaneous, short-lasting, and painful contractions of part of a muscle – can be stopped by stretching the muscle. Cramps occur in healthy individuals during and after exercise or sports, and when asleep. The muscles affected most frequently include the calves, knee flexors, and foot muscles. Tongue muscles may cramp after yawning.

Disorders of lower motor neuron cells (LMN) and motor neuropathies may cause cramps of all afflicted muscles. These pathological cramps do not occur in pure pyramidal or corticobulbar lesions. Cramps may occur in various myopathies (Table 2).

There is no evidence-based treatment for muscle cramps. Quinine derivates can be considered in individual cases but side effects must be taken into account.

Myotonia

Myotonia is sustained contraction and delayed relaxation of skeletal muscle caused by repetitive waxing and waning discharges of the muscle membrane. These give a characteristic electromyography (EMG) sound resembling a motorbike being started, previously called "dive bomber sound". Myotonia originates

Table 2. Myopathies with cramps and cramp-like symptoms

- Muscular dystrophies (e.g., BMD, LGMD1C, LGMD2A, LGMD2I)
- Metabolic myopathies: McArdle disease
- Thyroid myopathy
- Toxic myopathies; e.g., usage of diuretics (rarely: through hypocalcemia and hypomagnesemia), pyridostigmine (myasthenia gravis), statins (autoimmune necrotizing myopathy), zidovudine (exercise-induced myalgia)
- DM types 1 and 2 (usually not painful)
- Nondystrophic myotonias: usually myotonia is not painful except in sodium channel myotonias
- Brody disease, sarcoplasmic reticulum Ca^{2+}ATPase deficiency causes delayed muscle relaxation and silent cramps with stiffness as prominent complaint. Onset is usually in the first decade, but can be in adolescence
- Idiopathic

Muscle cramps can also occur:
- In the third trimester of pregnancy
- Following strenuous exercise
- With disturbed metabolism: hypomagnesemia, hypocalcemia (exclude vitamin D deficiency), hypothyroidism, renal or liver dysfunction

from the muscle and – in contrast to muscle cramps – occurs spontaneously without stimulation of the muscle through a nerve action potential. Action myotonia (Video 1) is slow relaxation of a muscle after voluntary contraction. Percussion myotonia occurs after mechanical stimulation of a muscle with a reflex hammer. Patients may complain of loss of relaxation when shaking hands, after grasping objects, or when playing the piano or organ. Repeated contraction decreases myotonia in DM types 1 and 2. Increased myotonia after repeated contractions and cold-induced myotonia are features of paramyotonia congenita.

Pain in neuromuscular diseases

Neuropathic pain must be distinguished from musculo-skeletal pain resulting from contractures, overuse, or inflammation. Neuropathic pain can be localized in the area of an affected nerve or nerve root and may be more often present at rest, especially at night. Neuropathic pain and other exteroceptive system symptoms usually occur in diabetic, alcoholic, and amyloid neuropathy. Acute radicular pain is a feature of Lyme radiculoneuritis. Various types of pain can be present in or even precede weakness in GBS.

Muscle pain at rest may occur in dermatomyositis, polymyositis, viral myositis, and rhabdomyolysis. Stiffness can be an accompanying feature. Pain during exercise occurs in McArdle disease. Muscle pain can also be found in muscular dystrophies; for example, facioscapulohumeral dystrophy (FSHD), Becker

muscular dystrophy (BMD), and limb girdle muscular dystrophy (LGMD) type 2I.

Fasciculations and myokymia

"Muscle twitches," or fasciculations, are spontaneous simultaneous contractions of all muscle fibers belonging to a single motor unit. The number of muscle fibers per motor unit varies from six in the thenar muscle to 600 in the gastrocnemius muscle. As a consequence, the type of fasciculation can vary between fine and coarse. Fasciculations do not result in coordinated movement of a muscle. Sometimes patients with fasciculations complain of restlessness in the muscles or of a feeling of ants creeping under the skin, but usually fasciculations pass unnoticed. To interpret fasciculations, the muscle must be examined at rest. Fasciculations can increase following strenuous contraction or after tapping the muscle. In healthy individuals, fasciculations may occur in various muscles including the calves and knee flexors following strenuous exercise and sports (Video 2). Treatment of myasthenia gravis with pyridostigmine may induce fasciculations (Video 3). Fasciculations together with muscle cramps may be a harbinger of motor neuron disease (MND)/ALS, or be an innocent but sometimes incapacitating affliction (Table 3).

Diseases that affect peripheral innervation may cause fasciculations. Reinnervation will lead to larger motor units and to coarse fasciculations (Video 4). Waves of fasciculations and of myokymia may mimic undulations. Undulating myokymia is a feature of neuromyotonia (Isaac's syndrome, Morvan's syndrome; Video 5) and of

Table 3. Neuromuscular disease that may manifest with cramps and fasciculation

- ALS: usually widespread EMG abnormalities; fasciculations, spontaneous muscle fiber activity, and neurogenic MUPs
- Progressive muscular atrophy: may be present as antecedent features for 1–2 yr
- Kennedy disease: usually more signs on careful examination; e.g., gynecomastia, postural tremor
- Late-onset SMA III, SMA IV, siblings of patients with spinal muscular atrophy, carrying homozygous deletions of SMN1 genes
- CMT 2
- Multifocal neuropathy: affected muscles are also weak
- Peripheral nerve hyperexcitability syndromes: Morvan's and Isaac's syndromes
- Treatment with gold salts
- Familial occurrence with autosomal dominant (AD) inheritance and electrophysiological signs of polyneuropathy
- Idiopathic muscle cramp–myalgia–fasciculation syndrome

- Cramps and fasciculation in the calves and posterior muscles of the lower legs occur in healthy persons; by definition, EMG may show fasciculation but no signs of denervation activity
- There is moderate quality evidence that quinine significantly reduces cramp frequency, intensity, and cramp days in dosages between 200 and 500 mg/day. There is less evidence for efficacy of vitamin B complex, naftidrofuryl, and calcium-channel blockers such as diltiazem in the management of muscle cramps (Level C)

rippling muscle disease. Fasciculation is not a feature of myopathy.

Myokymia, the term applied to spontaneous rhythmic and transient movements of a few muscle bundles within a muscle, does not cause movement in a joint. Myokymia may occur in healthy persons after strenuous exercise. Well known is myokymia in the orbicularis oculi muscle, which is associated with fatigue. Waves of myokymia are a feature of peripheral nerve hyperexcitability syndrome.

Atrophy and pseudohypertrophy

The volume of a skeletal muscle is determined by genetic predisposition, nutritional state, activity, and exercise. Unfortunately, no clear definitions exist for hypertrophy or atrophy in an individual patient. In severely ill patients and after a period of inactivity, generalized muscle atrophy occurs. Generalized atrophy can even occur after a period of two weeks of bed rest. In these patients, the skeletal muscle biopsy shows type 2 muscle fiber atrophy. Following denervation, atrophy of the corresponding muscle is noted after two weeks (Figure 1). Hypertrophy of the calves can be a residual finding after chronic, long-standing reinnervation in GBS, or S1-radiculopathy (Figure 2), or Charcot–Marie–Tooth (CMT) disease. Hypertrophy of leg muscles is a feature of Becker myotonia. Pseudohypertrophy of the calves due to increase in fat and connective tissue may occur in Duchenne and Becker muscular dystrophies (Figure 3), and in some of the LGMD, including the sarcoglycanopathies, LGMD2C, LGMD2I, and LGMD2L.

Atrophy caused by long-standing functional denervation of the neuromuscular junction that is blocked and destroyed by antibodies, can be a residual feature of myasthenia gravis in remission and in anti-muscle-specific kinase (MuSK) myasthenia gravis. Bulbar muscles are frequently affected (Figure 4). Hypertrophy of the tongue, macroglossia, can occur in hypothyroidism, BMD, Pompe disease, and amyloid myopathy.

Hypotonia and hypertonia

Hypotonia is the loss of resistance during passive movement. Hypertonia is defined as increased resistance during passive movement and results from upper pyramidal tract lesions that cause loss of inhibition. Hypertonia is characterized by a velocity-dependent increase in tonic stretch reflexes with exaggerated reflexes resulting from hyperexcitability. A consequence of hypertonia is the loss of dexterity that can be observed in patients with unilateral or bilateral lesions of the pyramidal tract. Bilateral lesions of the corticobulbar tracts may cause difficulties with tongue movements (Video 6). Some of these patients may even lose the ability to protrude the tongue.

Weakness

Flaccid weakness is the predominant sign of most neuromuscular diseases. Bulbar weakness may cause nasal speech, if the soft palate is weak, or dysarthria, due to weak facial or tongue muscles, or dysphagia. Characteristic facies myopathica may evolve, if all facial muscles are weak. Mild arm or hand weakness is

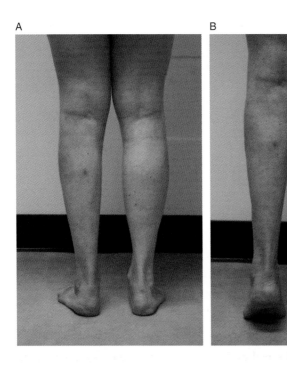

A   B

Figure 1. Atrophy of the left calf in a patient with S1 radiculopathy (A) becomes more marked as the patient stands on tiptoe (B). In that position – with hands on a desk or against a wall – the calf, biceps femoris, and semitendinosus muscles can be palpated.

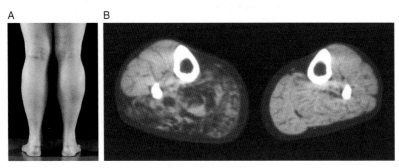

A   B

Figure 2. (A) Hypertrophy of the right calf in a patient with S1 radiculopathy. (B) Pseudohypertrophy becomes evident with CT scanning: abnormally thickened gastrocnemius and soleus muscles with areas of lower attenuation compatible with replacement of muscle by fat.

indicated by difficulties with daily tasks such as getting out of a chair, walking up/down stairs, carrying bags, or lifting objects out of cupboards. Mild leg weakness causes buckling of the knees or the tendency to trip. Symptoms resulting from specific weak muscles and corresponding diseases are summarized in Table 4.

For diagnostic purposes, muscle strength is measured using the Medical Research Council (MRC) grading system (Table 5). Manual muscle testing (MMT) using the MRC scale helps to evaluate the disease course and effect of treatment.

Sensory abnormalities

Pain and temperature senses and crude touch are conducted through the somatosensory exteroceptive system (Table 6). The numbers of nociceptors (receptors for pain) vary in different skin areas. Investigation

of temperature sensation is indicated only when small nerve fiber neuropathy is suspected. Sensorimotor neuropathy can be part of the spectra of DM and mitochondrial myopathy.

The somatosensory proprioceptive system for tactile sense, vibration sense, and motion and position senses is best examined using a wisp of cotton and the Rydel–Seiffer 128 Hz tuning fork for semiquantitative examination of the vibration sense.

Many patients with impaired proprioception also have a postural and kinetic tremor. A patient with severely impaired proprioception will develop sensory ataxia (Table 7), impaired tandem walking, and a positive Romberg sign. Even instability of the trunk can be observed when the patient comes to sit from a supine position. These patients may report difficulties with performing movements as weakness.

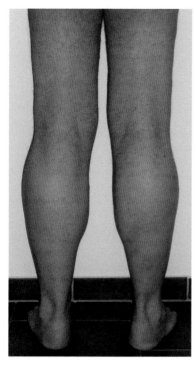

Figure 3. Hypertrophy of the calves in a patient with Becker muscular dystrophy.

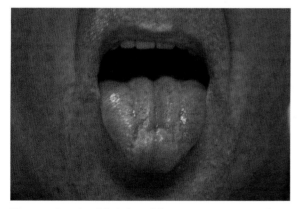

Figure 4. Atrophy of the edges of the tongue in a patient with classic myasthenia gravis.

Sensation is normal in motor neuron disorders, neuromuscular transmission disorders, and most myopathies.

Reflexes

Hyperreflexia results from hyperexcitability of the muscle stretch reflexes. If there is an abnormality of the muscle stretch – deep – reflexes, the response is manifested by either hypoactivity or hyperactivity; hypoactvity meaning diminution or absence of reflexes. Hyperactivity signifies varying degrees of increased speed and vigor of response, brisk reflexes, exaggeration of the range of movement, decrease in threshold, extension of the reflexogenic zone, and clonus. Hyporeflexia and areflexia result from lesions of part of the reflex arch, the afferent, efferent, or both. Weak skeletal muscles generate reduced or absent reflexes, ALS patients being an exception.

The jaw – masseter – reflex is usually hypoactive or absent, but is hyperactive in bilateral supranuclear lesions, which occur in ALS. Other pseudobulbar reflexes are the corneomandibular, and snout and palmomental reflexes. Elderly patients may have concomitant cerebovascular disease that can explain, through multiple small cerebral infarcts, the occurrence of snout and palmomental reflexes. Pseudobulbar affect – forced laughter, crying, and yawning – may be more reliable pseudobulbar signs.

A Hoffmann sign – opposition and flexion of the thumb and flexion of the index finger when tapping the nail or fingertip of the middle finger – suggests pyramidal tract involvement proximal to C8. The Hoffmann sign is clinically significant if asymmetric or very active.

Two grading systems for muscle tendon reflexes have been widely accepted. First, the Mayo Clinic scale is a nine-point ordinal scale grading reflexes from −4 (absent) to +4 (persistent clonus), 0 being normal. Second, the NINDS myotatic reflex scale grades reflexes from 0 (absent) to 4 (enhanced including clonus). Interobserver agreement on the two scoring systems, however, is poor and a verbal description of reflexes is often more useful. Asymmetry of muscle stretch reflexes and discrepancy between briskness of reflexes between the bulbar region, and arms or legs raise suspicion of a pathological condition. Relatively normal Achilles tendon reflexes with absent knee jerks can be seen in muscular dystrophies.

Superficial abdominal reflexes are frequently intact in corticospinal tract disease. The Babinski sign, the extensor plantar response, represents an inversion of the normal plantar response – plantar flexion of the toes – that is elicited by stimulation of the lateral plantar surface of the foot with a blunt point.

Autonomic functions

History taking identifies complaints of irregular heart action, orthostatic hypotension, increased or decreased

Table 4. Muscle weakness, symptoms, and associated neuromuscular diseases

Muscles affected	Symptoms	Examples of diseases
External ocular muscles	Diplopia, blurred vision	Miller–Fisher syndrome (MFS, Video 8): early Guillain–Barré syndrome (GBS) Diabetes mellitus (acute: usually one cranial nerve) Myasthenia gravis (fluctuating) Congenital myasthenia gravis Lambert–Eaton myasthenic syndrome (LEMS): late Oculopharyngeal muscular dystrophy (OPMD): usually no diplopia perceived by the patient Myotonic dystrophy (DM) type 1 (ptosis prominent): usually no diplopia perceived by the patient Mitochondrial cytopathy (often not perceived by the patient due to the chronic progressive nature: chronic progressive external ophthalmoplegia (CPEO); Figure 11)
Eyelid (levator palpebrae muscle)	Ptosis Functional blindness Neck pain from increased backward position of the head	Myasthenia gravis (asymmetric); patient may wear sunglasses LEMS (late) OPMD DM type 1 Mitochondrial cytopathy (in early phase, asymmetric) Pompe disease Beware that rigid contact lenses may cause ptosis
Muscles for mastication	Slow, impaired mastication (patient supports the jaw with one hand)	Amyotrophic lateral sclerosis (ALS) Kennedy disease Myasthenia gravis Anti-MuSK myasthenia gravis OPMD DM type 1 Congenital myopathy
Facial muscles	Sleeping with eyes open Loss of facial expression: asymmetry at rest, when speaking or laughing Hollow temples Drooling Difficulty whistling, drinking through straw, blowing up a balloon Biting on cheeks	GBS Lyme radiculoneuritis Myasthenia gravis Anti-MuSK myasthenia gravis Congenital myasthenia gravis Facioscapulohumeral dystrophy (FSHD) (Figure 12) Congenital myopathy OPMD Myotonic dystrophy type 1 (Figure 13) Proximal myotonic myopathy (PROMM, DM type 2: not as prominent as in DM type 1) Mitochondrial cytopathy
Muscles for swallowing	Dysphagia Change of diet Weight loss (>10% is concerning)	ALS Progressive muscular atrophy (PMA – late in disease) Kennedy disease GBS and MFS Myasthenia gravis Anti-MuSK myasthenia gravis LEMS OPMD Sporadic inclusion body myositis (sIBM) Myositis DM type 1
Muscles for phonation and articulation	Dysarthria: slurred speech, nasal speech Soft speech: limp, falling, and nonmoving palate Hoarse speech	ALS Kennedy disease Myasthenia gravis Anti-MuSK myasthenia gravis OPMD DM type 1 Charcot–Marie–Tooth (CMT) disease type 2A Hereditary neuralgic amyotrophy
Tongue	Dysphagia, dysarthria	ALS and PMA Kennedy disease Myasthenia gravis DM type 1
Muscles of the neck	Neck pain	ALS and PMA Myasthenia gravis

Table 4. (cont.)

Muscles affected	Symptoms	Examples of diseases
	Patients may actively stabilize the head by supporting the chin Head drop Difficult head fixation when rising from supine position	Anti-MuSK myasthenia gravis FSHD DM type 1 sIBM Myositis Idiopathic dropped head syndrome
Muscles of the shoulders and upper arms	Heavy feeling Difficulty washing hair, brushing teeth Difficulty taking objects down from shelves	Motor neuron diseases (asymmetry in ALS and PMA) Spinal muscular atrophy (SMA) types 3 and 4 Myasthenia gravis Anti-MuSK myasthenia gravis LEMS Most muscular dystrophies (asymmetry in FSHD; Figure 14) Pompe disease Myositis
Muscles of lower arms and hands	Difficulty writing or using PC, handling objects, fastening buttons Difficulty carrying shopping bag (finger flexor muscles)	ALS and PMA (asymmetry) Multifocal motor neuropathy (MMN – asymmetry) Neuropathies Distal myopathies DM type 1 sIBM (deep finger flexor muscles)
Muscles of the pelvis and upper legs	Difficulty rising from chair and from squatting position Difficulty climbing stairs Loss of running ability Waddling gait	ALS and PMA (asymmetry) Kennedy disease SMA types 3 and 4 GBS and chronic inflammatory demyelinating polyneuropathy (CIDP) LEMS Most muscular dystrophies and other myopathies In Becker muscular dystrophy (BMD) and IBM the quadriceps femoris muscle can be the first symptomatic muscle
Muscles of the lower legs and feet	Tripping over Foot drop Pushing off	ALS and PMA (asymmetric) MMN (asymmetric) All motor neuropathies FSHD (asymmetric) Distal myopathies OPMD DM type 1 Myofibrillar myopathies Sporadic IBM Sarcoid myopathy
Paraspinal muscles	Tiredness in the back Bent spine Scoliosis Loss of upright posture	ALS and PMA FSHD Central core disease Myositis Pompe disease OPMD sIBM Dermatomyositis and polymyositis Bent spine syndrome Axial myopathy (Video 9)
Abdominal wall muscles	Drooping abdomen	Pompe disease FSHD
Respiratory muscles	Dyspnea Morning headaches Nightmares Orthopnea Postural drop → >10% decrease in forced vital capacity in supine position compared with sitting position	ALS and PMA SMA type 3 GBS (early) CIDP (late) Myasthenia gravis BMD (late) FSHD (late) Myotonic dystrophy Congenital myopathies Bethlem myopathy Pompe disease Myofibrillar myopathies

Note. Dysarthria due to muscle weakness: nasal speech with weak palate; hollow vowels and consonants (especially "G" and "C", explosive pronunciation of "P" and "B"). Spastic speech is monotonous and slow.

Table 5. Medical Research Council scale for assessment of muscle strength

Grade 0	No contraction
Grade 1	Flicker or trace of contraction
Grade 2	Active movement, with gravity eliminated
Grade 3	Active movement against gravity
Grade 4	Active movement against gravity and resistance
Grade 5	Normal power

The MRC scale represents an ordinal scale. Compared with measurements that express strength in Newtons, most muscle power is measured as MRC grade 4–5. Only a minor part of the range of power reflects grades 0–4. There is a large interobserver but small intraobserver variation. Extension of the MRC scale with grades 4–5 can be useful. Other refinements of the scale (MRC 3–4, 4+, 5–) add little diagnostic value.

Recent research using the Rash technique indicated that a more simplified version of the MRC scale with only four modalities (0: paralysis; 1: severe weakness; 2: slight weakness; 3: normal strength) is more reliable to measure strength in patients with immune-mediated neuropathies and Pompe disease.

Table 6. Evaluation of the somatosensory system

	Nerve fibers	Qualities	Symptoms	Examination
Exteroceptive system (vital sensation)	Small myelinated or unmyelinated: slow conducting	Pain Temperature Crude touch	Neuropathic pain Analgesia Hypalgesia Hyperalgesia Disturbed temperature sense	Sharp point Two-point discrimination
Proprioceptive system (gnostic sensation)	Large myelinated fibers with thick myelin sheaths: fast conducting	Tactile sense Vibration sense	Numbness Tremor Loss of coordinated movements Postural instability	Wisp of cotton Rydel–Seiffer tuning fork (128 Hz) Fingertip–nose test Romberg test Tandem walking

- Neuropathic pain can be burning, aching, or lancinating
- Complaints of too cold or warm feet or hands, and loss of adaptation to temperature changes are often very incapacitating
- Analysis of temperature sense is usually cumbersome in the consultation room
- Anesthesia, hypesthesia, hyperesthesia are aspecific terms
- Paresthesias are abnormal spontaneous sensations in the absence of specific stimulation: feelings of cold, warmth, numbness, tingling, crawling, heaviness, compression, and itching
- Dysesthesias: distorted, usually painful or electric sensations after tactile or painful stimulation
- Tandem walking: ask the patient to walk along an imaginary straight line with eyes open placing one heel directly in front of the toes of the other foot. Observe if the patient remains stable when turning around rapidly

Table 7. Diseases with sensory ataxic neuropathy as the accompanying or predominant feature

- Kennedy disease
- Miller–Fisher syndrome
- Sensory and sensorimotor variants of chronic inflammatory demyelinating neuropathy
- Paraneoplastic sensory neuronopathy
- Neuropathy associated with IgM gammopathy
- Sensory ataxic neuropathy caused by mutations of the mitochondrial gene for polymerase gamma 1 (POLG1): SANDO syndrome (sensory ataxic neuropathy, dysarthria, ophthalmoplegia)
- Some forms of spinocerebellar ataxia (e.g., SCA17)

See also Table 22.1.

sweating, gastrointestinal motility dysfunction, impaired micturition, and male erection dysfunction. Orthostatic hypotension is defined as a decrease in systolic blood pressure of over 20 mmHg and/or a decrease in diastolic pressure of 10 mmHg, three minutes after rising from a supine position. Autonomic dysfunction can be prominent in GBS and other neuropathies (diabetes mellitus and other metabolic diseases, alcohol abuse, paraneoplastic primary amyloidosis), DM type 1, and mitochondrial cytopathy.

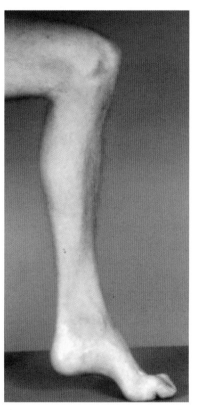

Figure 5. Pes equinovarus in a patient with CMT1A.

Musculoskeletal abnormalities

Disuse of the joints in chronic neuropathy and myopathy may result in contractures and deformity such as clawing of the toes, pes cavus, and pes equinovarus (Figure 5). Weakness of the shoulder muscles causes a frozen shoulder with pain and loss of function of the arm. Winging of the scapula will severely impair abduction of the arm further than 30° as the deltoid muscle cannot function with a loose scapula.

Contractures that are not related to muscle weakness are a feature of Bethlem myopathy (Figure 6). Examples are contractures of the fingers, elbow, Achilles tendon, and torticollis in Bethlem myopathy and of the Achilles tendon, elbow, and posterior cervical muscles (rigid neck) in Emery–Dreifuss muscular dystrophy. Later on in both diseases, limited forward flexion of the thoracic and lumbar spine (rigid spine) may occur.

Abnormalities of posture including scoliosis indicate an onset of a neuromuscular disease before cessation of normal growth. Increased lumbar lordosis may result from weak paraspinal and pelvic muscles; for example, in BMD (Video 7). Increased thoracic kyphosis is the result of weak paraspinal thoracic muscles as seen, for example, in survivors of poliomyelitis. Both postural abnormalities occur in ALS, progressive muscular atrophy (PMA), and Pompe disease. Hyperlaxity can be found in patients with Bethlem and Ullrich myopathies and occasionally in patients with congenital myopathy.

Neuromuscular manifestations are frequently part of a systemic disease (Table 8). Alternatively, in some diseases, other organs and tissues may also be affected; for example, the occurrence of cataracts before the age of 50 years in DM, stroke in mitochondrial cytopathy, gastrointestinal symptoms in DM type 1, and skin abnormalities in dermatomyositis.

A

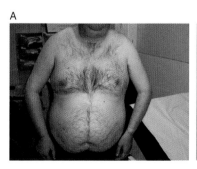

B

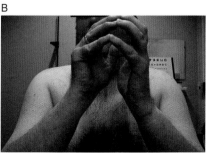

Figure 6. Contractures of the elbows (A) and of the finger flexors (B) in a patient with Bethlem myopathy.

Table 8. Examples of neuromuscular syndromes in systemic diseases

- Neuropathy in diabetes mellitus and other metabolic diseases (e.g., renal insufficiency)
- Vasculitic neuropathy in polyarteritis nodosa, Wegener's disease, and other diseases with systemic vasculitis
- Paraneoplastic neuropathy
- Neuropathy in primary amyloidosis (associated with hematological malignancy)
- Critical illness polyneuropathy
- Critical illness myopathy
- Dermatomyositis and polymyositis in the context of connective tissue disorders or malignancy
- Myopathy and neuropathy in hypothyroidism
- Thyreotoxic periodic paralysis
- Hypokalemic paralysis in renal disorders (both in proximal and distal renal tubular acidosis). Familial Gitelman syndrome, salt-losing tubulopathy, with hypokalemia and hypomagnesemia may manifest with proximal weakness in young adults
- Drug-induced neuropathy and myopathy

Cardiac function must be evaluated carefully in patients with muscular dystrophy, including BMD, LGMD 2I, Emery–Dreifuss muscular dystrophies, DM types 1 and 2, and mitochondrial cytopathy. Cardiac conduction abnormalities leading to arrhythmia may occur in the progressive and stationary phases of GBS.

Up to 10% of BMD patients have psychomotor retardation. Cognitive decline occurs in DM. In ALS patients, 30%–50% have some frontal dysfunction, and up to 10% of these have overt frontotemporal dementia.

Examination of a patient with a suspected neuromuscular disease

General remarks

A wide range of neuromuscular syndromes is recognized (Table 9). Some characteristic signs suggest one or more neuromuscular diseases (Table 10). The clinical examination starts with observing the patient rising from the chair in the waiting room and walking toward the consultation room. While listening to the history, dysarthria will become evident. The manner and speed of undressing illustrates how signs hamper that activity of daily life. History taking is aimed at unraveling a distinct pattern of complaints (Table 9). The family history may help to provide a rapid diagnosis if a hereditary neuromuscular disease is suspected.

General physical examination

The presence of cardiomyopathy, respiratory insufficiency (Table 11), autonomic failure, arthritis and other skeletal abnormalities, and skin changes or alopecia must be evaluated. The ophthalmologist can establish the presence of a cataract in DM type 1 and type 2, and of retinitis pigmentosa in mitochondrial disease.

Neurological examination

Table 12 gives tips for examining patients with a possible neuromuscular disease. One is advised to examine specifically those parts of the nervous and skeletal muscle systems that are likely to be affected; for example, the legs in a patient with diabetes who could have neuropathy.

Very elaborate examination of the sensory system is usually not necessary if a diagnosis like ALS, myasthenia gravis, or Pompe disease is considered. Patients with Kennedy disease may have sensory neuropathy. Cognition and mental development are assessed if indicated.

Examination of the head and neck, and cranial nerves

Physiological anisocoria of the pupils with a diameter difference of up to 1 mm occurs in 5%–10% of healthy persons. Responses to light and accommodation speed/ability must be reported. Ptosis, ocular movements, and gaze are rapidly assessed. If necessary, provocation tests are done (see also Table 34.1).

The soft palate, tongue, and facial muscles are inspected at rest and during activity. Slight weakness of the orbicularis oculi muscle leaves the eyelashes visible when closing the eye. If the weakness is greater, the sclera can be seen or even Bell's phenomenon; that is,

Table 9. Common neuromuscular syndromes

Syndrome	Signs	Causes	Remarks
Axonal polyneuropathy: i.e., more or less symmetric loss of sensation, less prominent motor findings Distal more than proximal Legs more affected compared with arms	No walking on heels Foot drop If severe: steppage gait	CMT Diabetes mellitus Vitamin B1 deficiency Alcohol Idiopathic Vasculitits	Pain may be prominent Reflexes in the legs can be absent In most variants of CMT motor > sensory signs Consider demyelinating neuropathy if arm reflexes are absent
Limb girdle syndrome: i.e., more or less symmetric weakness of proximal muscles of pelvis and upper legs Weakness of shoulders and upper arms less prominent	Patient cannot rise from deep chair without help of arms, or climb stairs without holding the railings Gowers' sign (Video 7) Waddling gait (Video 7)	Kennedy disease SMA types 3 and 4 LEMS BMD LGMDs Pompe disease DM type 2 Myositis Hypothyroid myopathy	Hip and knee flexor and foot extensor muscles affected early due to physiologically less reserve capacity of muscles Hip extensor, adductor, and abductor muscles of leg, and foot flexor muscles stronger If reflexes absent and no skeletal muscle atrophy, consider motor variant of CIDP
Prominent bulbar weakness without diplopia	Dysphagia leading to weight loss and aspiration Dysarthria	ALS and PMA Kennedy disease Myasthenia gravis Anti-MuSK myasthenia gravis Mitochondrial cytopathy OPMD DM type 1	Patients with Kennedy disease also have limb girdle weakness and postural tremor Hyperreflexia in ALS Fluctuating weakness in myasthenia gravis
Prominent bulbar weakness with ptosis and diplopia	Dysphagia causing weight loss and aspiration Dysarthria	Myasthenia gravis Anti-MuSK myasthenia gravis	Ptosis and impaired ocular motility in mitochondrial myopathy, OPMD, and DM
Acute respiratory insufficiency	Rapidly progressive weakness and respiratory insufficiency Deterioration within days to a maximum of 4 wk	GBS ALS Myasthenia gravis	Less than 10% of patients with ALS and myasthenia gravis have onset with respiratory insufficiency
Slowly progressive asymmetric atrophy and weakness of hand muscles	Abnormalities suggest motor neuropathy Progression over months	MMN Focal SMA sIBM	No sensory signs Rarely leg onset sIBM: deep finger flexors weak
Facial weakness and winged scapula	Facies myopathica Eye closure incomplete No diplopia	FSHD	Asymmetry
Winged scapula	Usually increase in winging with forward extension of arms Increased winging with abduction of arms (weakness of trapezius muscle)	FSHD LGMD2A Pompe disease Spinal accessory nerve lesion	Asymmetry can be prominent
Rhabdomyolysis	Acute (hours–days) muscle pain and limb girdle pattern of weakness, dark urine, very high serum CK levels Spontaneous recovery in days–weeks	Excessive muscle activity (e.g., seizure) Crush, trauma Ischaemia Drugs (e.g., statins), toxins Hyperthermia Viral infection Myopathy, mainly metabolic and some muscular dystrophies	Myoglobinuria may cause potentially irreversible acute renal failure Statins are also associated with more gradual-onset necrotizing myopathy, which may persist after discontinuation of the statin and improve with immunosuppressive agents.

We did not aim to present a comprehensive survey of all neuromuscular syndromes as most of these will be discussed in individual Cases. Table 9 can help to rapidly recognize common neuromuscular syndromes.

Table 10. Characteristic signs that suggest one or more diseases

Sign	Disease	Remark
Cataract before age 50 yr	Myotonic dystrophy types 1 and 2	
Cardiac involvement (see also Table 38.1)	GBS DMD and BMD patients and carriers LGMD1B LGMD 1E LGMD 2D-F LGMD 2I Emery–Dreifuss MD (patients and carriers) Myofibrillar myopathies DM types 1 and 2	Isolated cardiomyopathies are excluded
Skin changes	POEMS syndrome Lyme radiculoneuritis Lepromatous neuropathy Vasculitic neuropathy Dermatomyositis	Not all features of POEMS syndrome are obligatory with the exception of the M-protein antecedent erythema migrans
Ptosis	MFS (with diplopia and ataxia) Myasthenia gravis (all forms) Mitochondrial cytopathy OPMD DM type 1 Pompe disease	Ptosis can be asymmetric in myasthenia gravis, mitochondrial cytopathy, and Pompe disease
Enlarged tongue	BMD Amyloid myopathy in primary amyloidosis Pompe disease Hypothyroidism	
Dropped head	ALS and PMA CIDP Myasthenia gravis Anti-MuSK myasthenia gravis Central core disease (a congenital myopathy) DM type 1 Mitochondrial cytopathy Dermatomyositis and polymyositis sIBM Idiopathic isolated neck extensor myopathy (axial myopathy)	Weakness of neck extensor muscles may cause dysphagia Abnormal flexor contraction in cervical dystonia causes pseudoextensor weakness
Perioral fasciculation	Kennedy disease (Video 10)	Rare in ALS
Percussion-induced rapid muscle contractions, mounding, and rippling	LGMD1C	
Deep finger flexor weakness	sIBM	
Elbow contracture (see also Table 42.1)	Emery–Dreifuss muscular dystrophy Desmin myopathy Bethlem myopathy	Wrist flexors, knee, and ankle contractures also occur
Proximal leg weakness and dry mouth	LEMS	LEMS patients with small-cell lung cancer have rapid progression and early bulbar signs
Asymmetric foot drop	ALS and PMA, focal SMA Hereditary neuropathy with liability to pressure palsy (HNPP) MMN FSHD sIBM Compression neuropathy Vasculitic neuropathy	Can be exercise-induced Muscle atrophy is not obligatory in early HNPP and MMN Vasculitic neuropathy is usually associated with acute onset and pain

Table 10. (cont.)

Sign	Disease	Remark
Sensory ataxia	MFS (with diplopia and ptosis) Sensory CIDP Paraneoplastic and nonparaneoplastic, immune- mediated ganglionopathy Polyneuropathy and IgM monoclonal gammopathy Mitochondrial disease with POLG1 gene mutation	
Postural and kinetic tremor	Kennedy disease SMA CMT Polyneuropathy and IgM monoclonal gammopathy	

Table 11. Neuromuscular disorders with early or prominent respiratory failure

- Amyotrophic lateral sclerosis/motor neuron disease
- Progressive muscular atrophy
- Guillain–Barré syndrome
- Chronic inflammatory demyelinating neuropathy (rare)
- Classic myasthenia gravis
- Botulism
- Dystrophinopathy (Duchenne and severe Becker muscular dystrophies)
- Facioscapulohumeral dystrophy (late)
- DM type 1, Curschmann–Steinert disease (late)
- Limb girdle muscular dystrophy type 2I, fukutin-related protein deficiency
- Desminopathy
- Bethlem myopathy (can be early)
- Congenital myopathies (severe cases, usually early onset)
- Glycogen storage disease type 2, Pompe disease
- Respiratory insufficiency caused by interstitial lung disease, myositis, polyarthritis, Raynaud phenomenon, and fever represent the antisynthetase syndrome that is associated with autoantibodies against aminoacyl-tRNA synthetases; e.g., anti-Jo-1. Myositis may precede lung disease

- Watch out for orthopnea
- Check for postural drop: decrease of vital capacity (VC) of 10% when supine compared with sitting position
- Botulism is an extremely rare acute paralytic illness caused by neurotoxin of *Clostridium botulinum* that blocks presynaptic nerve terminals of neuromuscular junction. Following gastrointestinal symptoms of food poisoning, patients may have dysphagia, ptosis and external ophthalmoplegia, proximal muscle weakness, and respiratory failure. Internal ophthalmoplegia is an autonomic sign. Some patients require artificial ventilation. If the patients receive supportive care, in time the synapse will be restored and recovery occurs. Repetitive nerve stimulation may show an incremental response (see Case 36)

upward rotation of the eye. The frontal muscle is inspected when looking upward or frowning. Special attention is paid to facial expression at rest and when laughing, whistling, and pouting the lips. Note that in FSHD, weakness can be very subtle and asymmetric (Figure 7). Weakness of the zygomaticus muscles causes a vertical smile that is often observed in myasthenia gravis and DM (Figure 8).

When the patient speaks, dysarthria and hoarseness can be judged. With nasal dysarthria, air escapes through the nose. Interobserver agreement on dysarthria is low. Deafness occurs in CMT disease type 4

Table 12. What to look for during the examination of a patient who might have a neuromuscular disorder

Walk, stand and rise, recumbent position

1. Walking pattern: look for waddling gait (Duchenne gait < bilateral gluteus medius muscle, usually with hyperlordosis from weak paraspinal muscles; Videos 7, 9), foot drop – may become more evident after walking 10 m, ataxia (tandem gait)

2. Posture: increased lumbar lordosis, prolapsed abdominal wall, scoliosis

3. Look for contractures (e.g., rigid spine)

4. Standing and walking on heels and toes

5. Rising from a chair or squatting position without using the arms (if not possible: Gowers'sign)

6. Stable while standing on one leg (bending to collateral side < weak ipsilateral gluteus medius muscle = Trendelenburg sign)

7. Rising from supine to sitting position without using the arms

8. Making a hollow back (active hyperlordosis) in prone position

9. Ask the patient to cough to get an impression of the pulmonary function

10. Ask the patient in supine position, lying flat, to come to sit without assistance of the arms

Head and shoulders

1. Ptosis of tarsalis muscle (Horner sign), or levator palpebrae muscle (does not diminish when looking upwards), uni- or bilateral

2. Facial weakness:
   - asymmetric nasolabial fold
   - ability to close the eyes completely
   - weak closure of the eyes when forced open
   - delayed opening of the tightly closed eylids (myotonia)
   - horizontal movements of the angles of the mouth when pouting the lips and smiling
   - ability to whistle

3. Inspection of the tongue at rest (atrophic ridge, fasciculations) and when licking the lips, and inspection of rapid lateral tongue movements

4. Inspection of movements of soft palate

5. Extensors of the head and neck: usually very strong; dropped head syndrome: the patient cannot hold the head upright

6. Flexor muscles of the head and neck: not as strong as extensor muscles. Test with head upright and with chin on the chest (flexor muscle may appear stronger in that position)

7. Scapular winging, uni- or bilateral. Arms forward: trapezius muscle; arms sideways: serratus anterior muscle. Also inspect frontal aspect: rising of the scapula above the shoulder line. Winging may increase when pressing the stretched arms against a hard surface (Figure 15).

8. Examine scapulohumeral rhythm (rotator cuff function), presence of frozen shoulder

9. Testing of the deltoid muscles – anterior and lateral parts: compare strength with pressure in upper and lower arms. If scapular winging present, compare strength of ipsilateral deltoid muscle with pressure at scapula

10. Do not forget to test the pectoralis major muscles (ask the patient to make a smashing movement)

Arms and legs

1. Search for atrophy

2. Assess the presence of fasciculations, of myotonia, and percussion-induced rapid contractions

3. Establish muscle tonus

4. Test presence of contractures (elbow, wrist, Achilles tendons)

5. Test presence of hyperlaxity (elbow, wrist, fingers)

6. Assess pattern of weakness: proximal, distal, general, specific muscles; e.g., deep finger flexor muscles, calf muscles (Video 11)

7. Pseudoweakness of finger extensor muscles (radial nerve); if finger abductor and adducor muscles are weak (ulnar nerve)

8. Opening the hands after (forcedly) making strong fists (myotonia: inspect slow relaxation of flexor muscles of fingers and wrists (Video 1)

9. Ask the patient in recumbent position to lift one stretched leg against resistance (Hoover test)

10. Test vibration senses using validated instruments such as the Rydell–Seifer 128 Hz tuning fork and a two-point discriminating device

11. Assess dexterity of hands and feet with the patient tapping rapidly on a hard surface for 5 s

12. Assess dexterity and ataxia – eyes closed – with the fingertip–nose, the fingertip–nose–fingertip (of the examiner) and with the knee–heel tests

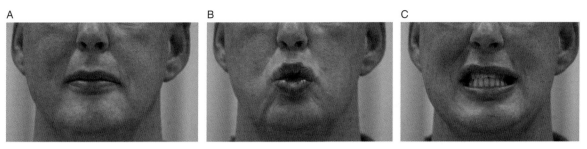

Figure 7. Subtle, asymmetric weakness of perioral muscles in a patient with facioscapulohumeral dystrophy. (A) Vertical nasolabial folds. (B) Some protrusion of the left lower lip and insufficient elevation of the left upper lip. (C) The width of the mouth does not change when the patient shows his teeth (compare with [A]).

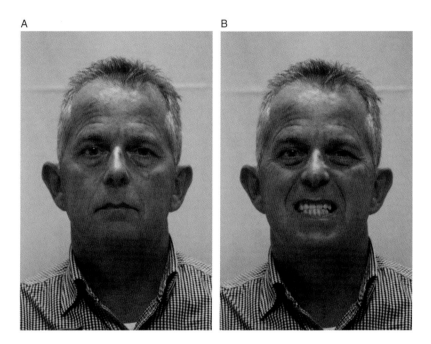

Figure 8. (A, B) Vertical smile in a patient with classic myasthenia gravis.

or Refsum disease, in X-linked CMT disease, and in mitochondrial cytopathy. Usually, analysis of taste and smell is of little value.

Atrophy of the temporal (Figure 9) and sternocleidomastoid muscles is a sign of DM type 1. The masseter reflex can be hyperactive in ALS.

Examination of the motor system

The patient's complaints are the starting point for choosing what to examine and to what extent. Owing to lack of time, not every muscle can be examined. The trophic situation of skeletal muscles, presence of fasciculation at rest, muscle tone, and muscle strength are evaluated. Table 13 summarizes main actions and innervation of the most important muscles. By examining passive movements of the limbs, one can

derive information about muscle tone and contractures.

Three examples of how to decide what to examine are:

- A progressive pseudobulbar syndrome raises suspicion of ALS. The tongue must be scrutinized at rest for fasciculation and atrophy, and when protruding for strength and rapidity of movements. Limb muscles are inspected for fasciculation, but only globally tested for proximal and distal weakness using the MRC scale (Table 5). It is usually not possible to examine every single muscle.
- If provocation tests of the orbicular and facial muscles reveal ptosis and diplopia, a diagnosis of myasthenia gravis will be established rapidly

15

A

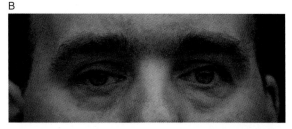

B

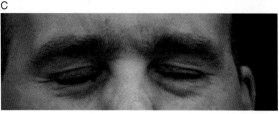

C

Figure 9. Patient with DM1. (A) Hollow temple caused by atrophy of the temporal muscle. (B) Mild ptosis. (C) Weakness of orbicularis oculi muscles leaves the eyelashes visible when the patient is asked to close the eyes firmly.

in a patient who complains of asymmetric, exercise-induced weakness of the limbs (see also Table 34.1).

- A patient with diabetes who complains of painful sensation on the soles of the feet and dizziness a few minutes after rising is likely to have diabetic sensory and autonomic neuropathy. Muscle testing focuses on muscles of the lower legs and feet, and of the hands.

Examination of the sensory system

The examiner decides to what extent the sensory system needs to be evaluated. It is best to start with examination of tactile sense over various areas of the body using a wisp of cotton. Pain sense can best be evaluated starting at the feet. If normal, a generalized neuropathy with involvement of small myelinated sensory fibers is unlikely. In this case, sharp–dull evaluation will add little value. Examination of temperature sense is not easy and is indicated only in suspected small fiber neuropathy.

The proprioceptive system can best be evaluated starting with the Rydell–Seiffer 128Hz tuning fork at the hallux. It is best to start the examination distally. If vibration is not perceived, or just for a split second, the examination must be extended to more proximal areas (midfoot, ankle, midtibia, knee, anterior superior process of the pelvic bone). If the patient feels the vibrations at the hallux for five seconds or longer, a generalized neuropathy with involvement of large myelinated sensory fibers is unlikely. If vibration sense is normal, evaluation of joint position and movement sense will add little diagnostic value.

Examination of reflexes

As a matter of routine, the biceps, triceps, brachioradial, knee, and ankle reflexes are examined. Depending upon what is found, the examination can be extended to search for other brisk reflexes or asymmetric reflexes for example, the trapezius, pectoralis major, deltoid, finger flexor and adductor reflexes, and for the Hoffman sign.

The abdominal skin reflexes are frequently absent in obese persons and after childbirth.

The soles of the feet are examined for a plantar response or Babinski sign that is usually accompanied by a triple response of the leg with flexion in the ankle, knee, and hip. If the Babinski sign is equivocal, stimulation of the lateral aspect of the foot with a blunt point is an alternative method of examining a dorsiflexion response of the toes (Chaddock sign, Video 4). Repeated stimulation may increase that response.

Examination of coordination

Tests of coordination such as the fingertip–nose or knee–heel tests and the Romberg test are indicated for the examination of sensory ataxia. The Romberg test is indicated to discriminate cerebellar from sensory ataxia. If the test is negative (i.e., no swinging) when the patient keeps the feet together, it can be helpful to repeat the test with the feet slightly apart. As the extensor and flexor muscles of the feet stabilize the legs while standing, the Romberg test is not useful in cases of mild lower limb weakness. Elderly and obese patients may find it difficult to keep the feet together.

Judgment about rapidity of alternate movements of nonweak muscles provides information about involvement of the pyramidal tracts. Disinhibition of reflexes due to pyramidal lesions causes alternating voluntary movements to be too slow, but they are usually regular.

Table 13. Main action and innervation of the most important muscles

Action	Muscle(s) involved	Nerve	Spinal segment
Test all muscles against resistance			
Shoulder and arm			
Elevation of shoulder	Trapezius	Spinal accessory nerve, C3, C4	C1, C2, C3, C4
Elevation and abduction of arm (arm sideways): fixation of scapula	Trapezius	Spinal accessory nerve, C3, C4	C1, C2, C3, C4
Pushing arm forward above the horizontal: fixation of scapula	Serratus anterior	Long thoracic nerve	C5, C6, C7
Pushing arm forward above the horizontal	Pectoralis major, clavicular head	Lateral pectoral nerve	C5, C6
Adduction of arm (pulls body upwards when climbing with arms fixed, throwing, pushing)	Pectoralis major, sternocostal head	Lateral and medial pectoral nerves	C6, C7
Adduction of arm (palpable when coughing; downstroke when swimming, rowing and climbing, hammering)	Latissimus dorsi	Thoracodorsal	C6, C7, C8
Abduction of upper arm 0°–30° 30°–180°	Supraspinatus Deltoid[a]	Suprascapular Axillary	C5, C6
External rotation of arm, elbow fixed against trunk (playing tennis, cello)	Infraspinatus	Suprascapular	C5, C6
Flexion of forearm	Forearm supinated: biceps brachii, brachialis Forearm midway: brachioradial	Musculocutaneus Radial	C5, C6
Extension of forearm	Triceps brachii	Radial	C6, C7
Supination of forearm	Supinator	Radial	C6, C7
Pronation of forearm; also flexion of forearm	Pronator	Median	C6, C7
Extension and abduction of hand (on radial side)	Extensor carpi radialis longus	Radial	C5, C6
Extension and adduction of hand (on ulnar side)	Extensor carpi ulnaris	Radial (posterior interosseus)	C7, C8
Flexion and abduction of hand (on radial side)	Flexor carpi radialis longus	Median	C6, C7
Flexion and adduction of hand (on ulnar side)	Flexor carpi ulnaris	Ulnar nerve	C7, C8, T1
Extension of fingers at metacarpophalangeal joints[b]	Extensor digitorum Thumb: extensor pollicis brevis	Radial (posterior interosseus)	C7, C8
Flexion of fingers at proximal interphalangeal joint	Flexor digitorum superficialis[c]	Median	C7, C8, T1
Flexion of distal phalanx of thumb	Flexor pollicus longus	Median	C7, C8
Abduction (upward movement) of thumb with back of hand on flat surface	Abductor pollicis brevis	Median	C8, T1
Opposition of thumb (toward little finger)	Opponens	Median	C8, T1
Abduction of little finger with back of the hand on flat surface	Abductor digiti minimi	Ulnar	C8, T1
Abduction of index finger with palm of hand on flat surface	First dorsal interosseus	Ulnar	C8, T1
Adduction of thumb toward palm of the hand	Adductor pollicis	Ulnar	C8, T1
Hip and leg			
Patient prone: heel to buttock	Hamstrings[d]	Sciatic	L5, S1, S2

17

Table 13. (cont.)

Action	Muscle(s) involved	Nerve	Spinal segment
Test all muscles against resistance			
Patient prone: extend flexed leg; alternative (patient supine): extend the leg with the limb flexed at the hip and the knee	Quadriceps femoris	Femoral	L2, L3, L4
Patient supine: flexion of thigh (advances limb during walking)	Iliopsoas aided by tensor fasciae latae	Femoral Superior gluteal	L1, L2, L3 L4, L5, S1
Patient supine: adduction of thigh	Adductors	Obturator	L2, L3, L4
Patient supine: abduction of thigh	Gluteus medius and minimus[e], Tensor fasciae latae	Superior gluteal	L4, L5, S1
Patient supine: extension of thigh (movement towards bench)[f]	Gluteus maximus Hamstrings	Inferior gluteal Sciatic	L5, S1, S2
Patient supine: dorsiflexion[g] of the foot; alternative: with knee flexed	Anterior tibial	Deep peroneal	L4, L5
Patient supine: inversion of the foot (inward dorsiflexion)	Posterior tibial	Tibial	L4, L5
Patient supine: eversion of the foot (outward dorsiflexion)	Peroneus longus and brevis	Superficial peroneal	L5, S1
Patient supine: dorsiflexion of the distal phalanx of the big toe/toes	Extensor hallucis/ digitorum longus	Deep peroneal	L5, S1
Patient supine: dorsiflexion of the toes	Flexor hallucis/digitorum longus	Tibial	L5, S1, S2
Patient supine: extension and plantar flexion of the foot	Gastrocnemius	Tibial	S1, S2
Patient supine with knee and hip flexed: plantarflexion of the foot	Soleus	Tibial	S1, S2

[a]Deltoid muscle also elevation and retraction of abducted arm; function hampered if supraspinatus muscle is paralyzed.
[b]Extensor digitorum longus and extensor pollicis longus muscles extend at interphalangeal joints; similar innervation and myelum segments as extensor digitorum and extensor pollicis muscles.
[c]Flexor digitorum profundus I and II muscles: flection of distal phalanx of index and middle fingers with proximal phalanx fixed (median nerve, C7, C8). Flexor digitorum III and IV muscles have the same function for ring and little finger (ulnar nerve, C7, C8). Deep finger flexor muscles are preferentially involved in IBM.
[d]Hamstrings: biceps femoris, semitendinosus, and semimembranosus muscles.
[e]Trendelenburg sign: when patient stands on one leg weak gluteus medius and minimus muscle lead to bending over to the other side.
[f]The gluteus maximus and hamstring muscles act together when walking, running, and climbing; the gluteus regulates flexion of hip when sitting down).
[g]Dorsiflexion of foot is synonymous with extension.

Provocation and function tests

Provocation tests can be indicated to reveal weakness in myasthenia gravis or myotonia (Video 1). If a patient complains of walking difficulties and the neurological examination gives no clear explanation, it is advised to observe the walking pattern over a short distance and while climbing a flight of stairs. There are a large number of functional scales, many disease specific, as in ALS or myasthenia gravis. Most are used for research purposes only.

Subsequent steps

After the history taking and neurological examination, most neuromuscular syndromes can be diagnosed. A normal neurological examination does not exclude a neuromuscular disease.

Laboratory tests and treatment strategies will be discussed in individual cases. Creatine kinase elevation of >10 upper limit of normal (ULN) usually excludes the neurogenic diseases spinal muscular atrophy (SMA), ALS, PMA and the neuropathies, Kennedy disease and the occasional case of late-onset SMA type 3 being a possible exception. In myopathy, CK activity can range from normal to highly elevated (>100 ULN). If CK activity is >10 ULN, EMG is rarely indicated as a myopathy is already suggested. Patients with normal CK, or CK <10 ULN, can have MND/ALS, neuropathy, myasthenia gravis, and myopathy.

Computer tomography (CT) or magnetic resonance imaging (MRI) is indicated for three reasons. First, imaging can detect abnormalities in clinically affected and unaffected muscles, plexus, or nerve roots. These include edema that MRI can demonstrate in myositis. Second, especially in research settings, MRI can help to follow disease progression and therapeutic efficacy. Third, a suitable muscle for biopsy can be selected. It should be kept in mind that in dystrophies, parts of muscle can be totally replaced by fat and connective tissue.

As many patients with myopathy have cardiological abnormalities, cardiac evaluation can be indicated (see also Table 38.1).

Electrophysiology

Electrophysiologal tests include EMG, repetitive nerve stimulation tests, single fiber EMG, and motor and sensory nerve conduction studies. The latter include analysis of late responses (F-waves and H-reflexes). These tests can be indicated for various reasons:

- To detect abnormalities if the clinical syndrome is ambiguous
- To discriminate between primary neurogenic and myopathic causes of disease
- To diagnose ALS and other motor neuron disorders

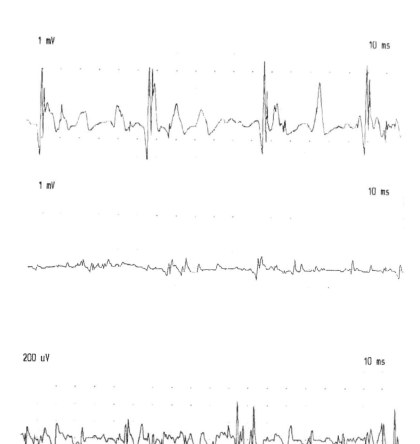

Figure 10. MUPs on needle EMG recording. Upper trace: neurogenic EMG. Maximal contraction elicits a markedly reduced interference pattern with one polyphasic and large amplitude MUP firing every 50 ms, implying a firing rate of 20 Hz. MUPs are large, due to collateral sprouting. The normal interference pattern is reduced because of loss of motor units.

Middle and lower traces: myopathic EMG. During moderate voluntary contraction many different, very small amplitude MUPs appear in a full interference pattern for most of the trace. This phenomenon is known as increased recruitment. Middle and upper traces have similar gains so that the difference between neurogenic and myopathic MUPs can be appreciated. The gain of the lower trace is increased in order to observe the many different, small MUPs. MUPs are small because each motor unit loses functional muscle fibers whereas the interference pattern is full because the number of motor units usually is not reduced in myopathy. Increased recruitment arises because a larger than normal number of motor units is required to produce moderate force.

A
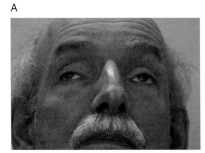

B
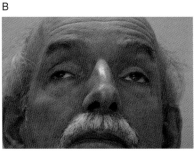

Figure 11. Bilateral ptosis and almost complete external ophthalmoplegia in a patient with mitochondrial cytopathy (A). When the patient tries to look upward, only the right eye abducts a little. The frontal muscle is not weak (B).

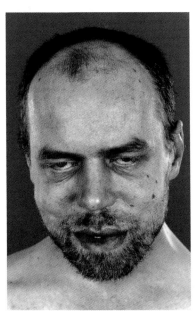

Figure 12. Almost complete loss of facial expression in a patient with FSHD who attempts to smile. The eyelids cannot be closed. The mouth is unsmiling.

- To discriminate between primary demyelinating and axonal neuropathy and thus characterize a neuropathy
- To demonstrate motor nerve conduction block
- To demonstrate abnormalities of proximal nerve conduction as can be demonstrated in radicular lesions and in many cases with chronic inflammatory demyelinating polyneuropathy (CIDP).
- To demonstrate dysfunction of neuromuscular transmission
- To detect dysfunction of the muscle membrane as in myotonia.

Needle EMG of bulbar, cervical, thoracic, and lumbosacral body regions will reveal the extent of the disease process in ALS and PMA. Needle EMG will usually help to differentiate between a neurogenic disorder and myopathy, but it should be kept in mind that spontaneous muscle fiber activity (fibrillations, positive sharp waves, and complex repetitive discharges) may occur in both neurogenic and myopathic disorders (Figure 10). For this reason, the older term "denervation potentials" can be ambiguous. The distinction between neurogenic and myopathic is made, therefore, by judging motor unit potentials (MUPs) during slight voluntary contraction. A typical neurogenic pattern is not full and shows few large, polyphasic, and giant MUPs. A typical myopathic pattern is full and shows many low amplitude MUPs. Especially in inclusion body myositis (IBM), however, a neurogenic pattern can be observed that may lead to confusion if the typical clinical picture is not taken into account.

Electromyographic abnormalities are not very helpful in diagnosing muscular dystrophies, myositis, or Pompe disease. Needle EMG can, however, be useful in patients with proximal weakness, in order to detect myotonia in DM type 2.

A change in evoked compound muscle action potential (CMAP) after repetitive motor nerve stimulation is an obligatory finding in a neuromuscular transmission disorder. Following 3 Hz stimulation, a decrease of the amplitude and area of the CMAP (decrement) will suggest dysfunction of postsynaptic neuromuscular transmission. Low amplitudes of CMAPs in patients with proximal weakness may suggest the Lambert–Eaton myasthenic syndrome (LEMS). Following repetitive 20 Hz stimulation, these low amplitudes will increase (increment), as can be explained by a presynaptic dysfunction of neuromuscular transmission.

Demonstration of motor nerve conduction block without widespread demyelination is indicative of multifocal motor neuropathy (MMN).

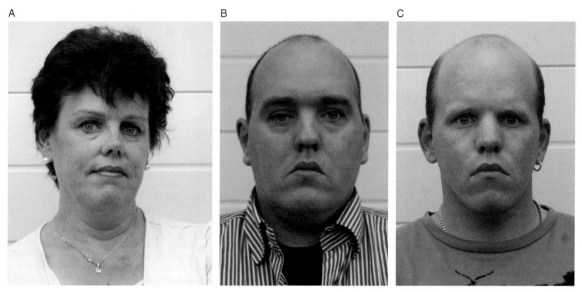

Figure 13. DM1. Three-generation family with anticipation. (A) 54-year-old woman with complaints of myotonia from the age of 30 years and progressive weakness since then. Hollow temples and atrophy of the sternocleidomastoid muscles. (B) 32-year-old son with frontal baldness, hollow temples, ptosis and unsmiling, "carp" mouth (also see Figure 9). (C) 28-year-old son without ptosis but with hollow temples, frontal baldness, and unsmiling mouth. Both men had onset during the first decade and psychomotor retardation. The maternal grandfather had cataracts removed at the age of 55 years. He died when 65 years old from cardiac arrest.

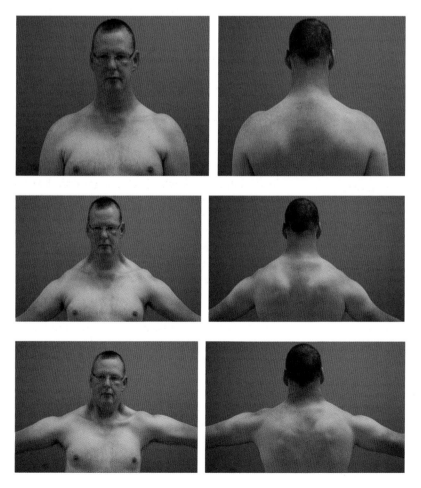

Figure 14. FSHD. Characteristic appearance of the shoulders. The trapezius muscle mounds up when the patient tries to abduct the arms. The shoulder blades slide upward and laterally. With great effort, the patient can keep the arms in the horizontal plane.

21

A 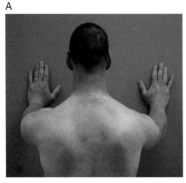 B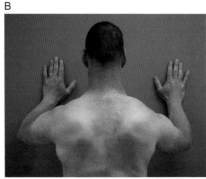

Figure 15. FSHD. Asymmetric winged scapulae. Asymmetry becomes more evident if the patient pushes the outstretched arms against a hard surface.

Suggested reading

Brooke MH. *A Clinician's View of Neuromuscular Diseases.* 2nd edn. Williams and Wilkins, Baltimore, MD, 1986.

Campbell W., ed. DeJong's *The Neurological Examination.* 6th edn. Lippincott Williams & Wilkins, Philadelphia, PA, 2005.

El-Tawil S, Al Musa T, Valli H, et al. Quinine for muscle cramps. *Cochrane Database Syst Rev* 2010; **12**: CD005044.

Gardner E, Gray DJ, O'Rahilly R. *Anatomy. A Regional Study of Human Structure.* 3rd edn. WB Saunders Company, Philadelphia, PA, 1969.

Gerable-Esposito P, Katzberg HD, Greenberg SA, et al. Immune-mediated necrotizing myopathy associated with statins. *Muscle Nerve* 2010; **41**: 185–190.

Guarantors of Brain. *Aids to the Examination of the Peripheral Nervous System.* Ballière Tindall, London, 1986.

Hiba B, Richard N, Hébert LJ, et al. Quantitative assessment of skeletal muscle degeneration in patients with myotonic dystrophy type I using MRI. *J Magn Res Imag* 2012; **35**: 678–685.

Huerta-Alardín AL, Varon J, Marik PE. Bench-to-bedside review: rhabdomyolysis – an overview for clinicians. *Critical Care* 2005; **9**: 158–169.

Jain KK. *Drug-Induced Neurological Disorders.* Hogrefe & Huber Publishers, Seattle, WA, 1996.

Katzberg HD, Khan AH, So YT. Assessment: symptomatic treatment for muscle cramps (an evidence-based review): report of the therapeutics and technology assessment subcommittee of the American academy of neurology. *Neurology* 2010; **74**: 691–696.

Kissani N, Mouttawakkil S, Chakib A, Slassi I. Fifteen cases of food-borne botulism in Morocco: significant diagnostic contribution of electrodiagnosis. *Rev Neurol* 2009; **165**: 1080–1085.

Manschot S, Van Passel L, Buskens E, et al. Mayo and NINDS scales for assessment of tendon reflexes: between observer agreement and implications for communication. *J Neurol Neurosurg Psychiatry* 1998; **64**; 253–255.

Merkies ISJ, Schmitz PIM, Van der Meché FGA, Van Doorn PA. Reliability and responsiveness of a graded tuning fork in immune mediated polyneuropathies. *J Neurol Neurosurg Psychiatry* 2000; 669–671.

Noback CR, Strominger NL, Demarest RJ, Ruggiero DA. *The Human Nervous System. Structure and Function.* 6th edn. Humana Press, Totowa, NJ, 2005.

Vanhoutte EK, Faber CG, Van Nes SI, et al. Modifying the medical research council grading system through Rasch analysis. *Brain* 2012; **135**: 1639–1649.

Classic amyotrophic lateral sclerosis: a retired bank manager with neck pain

Clinical history

While working is his garden, a 59-year-old man noticed pain in his neck and shoulders. He had some difficulty holding his head upright and could not rise easily from a squatting position. His GP referred him to a physical therapist with no effect. A neurologist performed an MRI scan of the cervical spine, which proved to be normal. As his CK activity was elevated and the EMG showed fibrillation potentials, myositis was suggested. On referral after six months, he also mentioned difficulty climbing stairs. When walking, he experienced cramps in the calves. In recent weeks, he had developed slurred speech and had problems fastening buttons. He had lost 10 kg (12% of his original weight). Pseudobulbar affect was not mentioned at the time.

Examination

Examination revealed pseudobulbar dysarthria, impressive atrophy of shoulder and arm muscles with widespread fasciculations (Figure 1.1), dropped head and bent spine caused by weak neck extensor muscles, MRC grade 3–4, and weak paraspinal muscles. In addition, he had mild atrophy of lower leg muscles. No fasciculations were noted in the legs.

Weakness of proximal arm muscles was more pronounced compared with distal weakness. He had bilateral foot drop. The masseter reflex and biceps brachii reflexes were hyperactive. His knee reflexes were normal and the Achilles tendon reflexes hypoactive. There was no Babinski sign. Sensation was normal. Lung vital capacity (VC) was 80% of that expected.

Ancillary investigations

CK activity was five times ULN. Needle EMG showed widespread spontaneous muscle fiber activity and neurogenic MUPs in arm, leg, and paraspinal muscles and fibrillations in the tongue. Motor nerve conduction was normal.

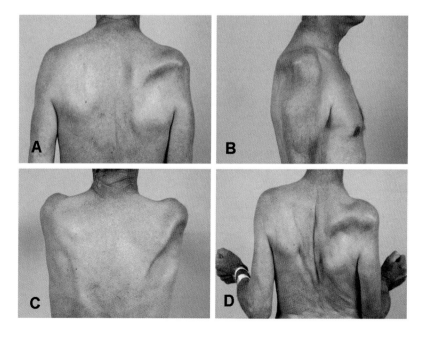

Figure 1.1. (A–D) Marked atrophy of the muscles of the right shoulder and upper arm and mild scapular winging. The supraspinatus, infraspinatus, and deltoid muscles have disappeared. The patient cannot elevate and abduct the right arm. The EMG showed denervation activity in muscles at the left side.

Diagnostic considerations

He had a progressive disease course with clinical signs of lower motor neuron (LMN) disease in the cervical, thoracic, and lumbosacral regions and upper motor neuron (UMN) signs in the bulbar and cervical regions. The former signs were atrophy, fasciculations, and weakness; the latter hypertonia, loss of dexterity, and hyperreflexia. This combination led to a diagnosis of amyotrophic lateral sclerosis (ALS, Table 1.1). Using the revised El Escorial Research Criteria for ALS (Table 1.2), he had definite ALS. Needle EMG confirmed the diagnosis of a diffuse neurogenic disease with normal motor nerve conduction, suggesting anterior horn cell dysfunction.

Table 1.1. Phenotypic classification of amyotrophic lateral sclerosis

Classic	M > F
Bulbar ~ 30%	F > M, older onset, ↓ prognosis
Flail arm, flail leg (very rare)	M > F, ↑ prognosis
Flail leg	
Respiratory	M > F, ↓ prognosis
UMN (pyramidal) predominant	younger onset, ↑ prognosis
Pure LMN (PMA)	M > F, younger onset, ↑ prognosis
Pure UMN (PLS)	younger onset, ↑ prognosis

Follow-up

He was treated with the anti-glutamate drug, riluzole. Eight months after onset, VC was 52% of what one would expect. For some time, he had complained of increased dyspnoea when supine. He had a decrease in VC of >10% when supine compared with the sitting position. This phenomenon of postural drop is caused by diaphragm weakness. As a consequence, VC must be tested in a sitting and lying position. Owing to dysphagia, he had progressive weight loss. A percutaneous endoscopic gastrostomy (PEG) was performed for parenteral feeding, but he died within weeks after the procedure.

General remarks

ALS/MND is by definition a severe, progressive disease with deterioration over a period of weeks to months. ALS forms part of a spectrum that encompasses primary lateral sclerosis (PLS), PMA, and ALS with or without frontotemporal dementia (FTD) (Figure 1.2). The annual incidence of ALS in the population older than 18 years is 2.4 per 100 000. The incidence is 2.2 in women and 3.1 in men (male: female incidence ratio = 1.4). The prevalence of ALS is about 6 per 100 000. The median age at onset is 60 years, and median time of survival is three years after symptom onset.

Table 1.2. Revised El Escorial Research Criteria for amyotrophic lateral sclerosis

Definite ALS
- LMN and UMN signs in three regions

Probable ALS
- LMN and UMN signs in two regions with at least some UMN signs rostral to LMN signs

Probable ALS (laboratory supported)
- LMN and UMN signs in one region or
- UMN signs in one or more regions
- Needle EMG abnormalities in at least two limbs. A muscle is considered abnormal if needle EMG shows both acute denervation (i.e., spontaneous muscle fiber activity) and chronic denervation (i.e., neurogenic MUPs). The cervical and lumbosacral regions require two abnormal muscles innervated by different nerves and roots

Possible ALS
- UMN and LMN signs in one region (together) or
- UMN signs in two or more regions
- UMN and LMN signs in two regions with no UMN signs rostral to LMN signs

These research criteria are widely used in the clinic.
UMN signs: hypertonia, loss of dexterity, clonus, Babinski sign, absent abdominal skin reflexes.
LMN signs: atrophy, weakness. If there is only fasciculation, search with EMG for active denervation.
Regions reflect neuronal pools: bulbar, cervical, thoracic, and lumbosacral.
Rostral: can reflect different regions (e.g., cervical and lumbosacral), or one region (e.g., in the cervical region, brisk biceps tendon reflex and atrophic and weak intrinsic hand muscles).

A

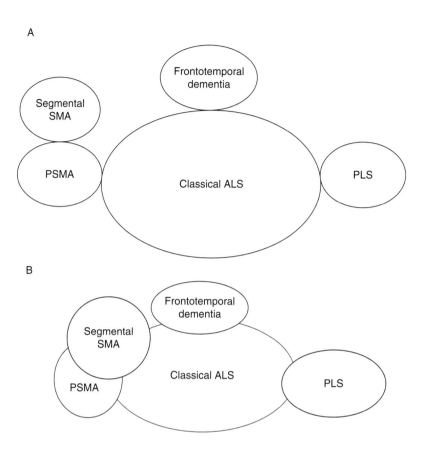

B

Figure 1.2. (A) T0: moot patients with motor neuron disease have classic amyotropic lateral sclerosis (ALS). Other syndromes include progressive spinal muscular atrophy (PSMA), segmental spinal muscular atrophy (SMA), frontotemporal dementia (FTD), and primary lateral sclerosis (PLS). (B) Three years after T0: about half of the patients with ALS will have died. Many patients with other motor neuron diseases will have developed ALS. Some patients with FTD develop overt signs of ALS.

Initially, ALS can be difficult to diagnose. Usually, ALS is diagnosed by exclusion. As a consequence of the healthcare system and cultural differences between countries, the mean time required to reach a diagnosis varies between 8 and 14 months after onset. Both patient's delay and doctor's delay explain the excessively long period until ALS is diagnosed in some cases.

Symptoms and signs of ALS are due to loss of UMN and LMN cells. In essence, ALS is characterized by a mixture of signs of flaccid and spastic paralysis, frequently in the same limb or in the bulbar region. Interestingly, these clinical phenotypes were strong prognostic factors, independent of age at onset and gender.

Diagnosis is difficult at an early stage as ALS can begin focally. Onset with asymmetric weakness is common in ALS. A foot drop suggests peroneal palsy or an L5 syndrome from a herniated lumbar disk. In an elderly patient, deltoid muscle weakness may cause a frozen shoulder pain syndrome that will be treated by a physical therapist for months. Many patients with bulbar-onset ALS are initially referred to an ENT-specialist for analysis of dysarthria and dysphagia.

Distinction between bulbar and pseudobulbar dysarthria is unreliable. In <5% of cases, patients may present with acute respiratory failure by selective involvement of phrenic motor neurons. Glottic narrowing due to vocal cord dysfunction may cause laryngospasm, stridor, and even sudden death. Active reflexes of weakened and atrophic muscles point to combined involvement of UMN and LMN cells (Video 4).

EMG helps to confirm clinical suspicion of LMN dysfunction, to detect signs of LMN dysfunction in clinically unaffected areas, and to diagnose ALS mimicking syndromes (Table 1.3). Some mimic syndromes reflect a treatable disease. Most have a much better prognosis.

ALS is considered to be a multifactorial disease. Complex genetic models take into account genetic variation in multiple genes as well as environmental and life-style factors that are more common in patients than in controls. These factors may have a disease-modifying effect with an increased or decreased risk of developing ALS. The best studied environmental factor that is associated with increased risk of ALS is cigarette smoking.

Table 1.3. Amyotrophic lateral sclerosis mimicking syndromes

Disease	Clinical features	Diagnostic test	Other
Cervical spondylotic myelopathy	Hyperreflexia and Babinski sign below region with weakness and atrophy; sensory signs Neurogenic bladder Slow progression (months–years)	Cervical MRI: stenosis and myelopathy EMG: LMN signs can be found in the cervical region	Respiration normal Coincidental MRI abnormalities in the elderly No firm evidence for benefit of surgery
sIBM	Initial symptoms: asymmetric weakness of quadriceps femoris, or of deep finger flexor muscles, or dysphagia Slow progression (months–years)	Muscle biopsy: rimmed vacuoles, endomysial mononuclear cell infiltrates and sometimes inclusion bodies EMG occasionally confusing as neurogenic MUPs can be found	Respiratory insufficiency: late Coincidental hyperreflexia in elderly people No curative treatment
MMN	Asymmetric weakness and atrophy of distal arm or hand muscles suggesting peripheral nerve dysfunction fasciculation No sensory loss Slow progression (months–years)	Electrophysiological evidence of motor nerve conduction block	MMN occurs in men between 20 and 60 years Respiration normal Good response to intravenous human immunoglobulins IVIg)
Kennedy disease (X-linked spinal and bulbar muscular atrophy)	Limb girdle weakness and atrophy Perioral fasciculation, dysphagia, respiratory insufficiency Sensory neuropathy, and postural tremor Gynecomastia in 50% of affected males Slow progression (years)	CAG repeat expansion in androgen receptor gene	Female carriers may have some weakness or muscle cramp–fasciculation syndrome
Other myelopathy syndromes: thoracic herniated disk, spinal dural arteriovenous fistula	Spastic legs No bulbar and upper limb signs Neurogenic bladder dysfunction, sensory signs Slow progression Acute deterioration (days–weeks) possible	MRI of the thoracic spine MR angiography if fistula suspected	Surgical treatment (prevention of spinal cord injury); embolization (fistula)
Primary progressive form of spinal multiple sclerosis (MS)	Spastic legs Disturbed proprioception Neurogenic bladder Slow progression (months–years)	Spinal cord and brain MRI cerebrospinal fluid (CSF) evidence of immunoglobulin synthesis	No curative treatment
Adult onset SMA type 4	Limb girdle weakness and muscle atrophy Fasciculation No UMN signs Slow progression (months–years)	Deletions of exons 7 and 8 in SMN gene	Slow progression Respiratory insufficiency: late

Early observational studies of Guam–ALS and experimental studies led to the suggestion of excitotoxicity and of oxidative stress as causative pathogenic mechanisms. These could act together. The neurotransmitter glutamate plays a central role in the excitotoxicity hypothesis. A relative excess of glutamate may cause too much neuronal stimulation, increased calcium influx, and consequent motor neuron cell damage. Scavenging of free oxygen radicals that emerge in this process may be insufficient.

Hereditary ALS

ALS shows familial occurrence in 5%–10% of patients. Inheritance is usually autosomal dominant. At least 16 genes of major effect are known to be associated with ALS. It is not clear whether all identified mutations are pathogenic. The most frequent ones, depending on geographical location, are C9ORF72, FUS, TARDBP, and copper/zinc superoxide dismutase 1 (SOD1). About one-fifth of familial ALS (FALS) cases have a mutation in the SOD1 gene on chromosome 21. Phenotypic variance does exist in cases of SOD1–FALS. More than 17 years after the identification of SOD1 as an ALS gene, the mechanisms of SOD1–FALS have still not been elucidated.

The distinction between FALS and sporadic ALS (SALS) has recently been challenged because of the breakthrough discovery of the C9ORF72 hexanucleotide repeat expansion in both FALS and SALS. Up to 60% of FALS cases can be explained by mutations in the C9ORF72 gene. Up to 10% of SALS carry this mutation. The frequency is dependent on geographical location and appears to be highest in Scandinavia, the apparent origin of the founder mutation. As a consequence, the exact meaning of a C9ORF72 mutation in SALS is not totally clear at present. The exact penetrance of C9ORF72 mutations is unknown, and as yet there are no publications on unaffected carriers of this mutation. Recently, a clinical algorithm was proposed, based on a positive family history of ALS or FTD and on the presence of cognitive or behavioral impairments of the patient. Patients who do not have a positive family history for FTD or ALS, and do not have cognitive or behavioral impairment, do not appear to carry C9ORF72 mutations. This emphasizes the point that to achieve a meaningful distinction of FALS versus SALS, one has to take into account the presence of FTD or cognitive and behavioral problems.

Recognizable phenotypes have been reported for some known mutations; for example, the A4V variant in SOD1, which produces a rapidly progressive primarily LMN syndrome. Mutations in FUS cause a young-onset, primarily LMN syndrome. The C9ORF72 hexanucleotide repeat expansion has a characteristic phenotype with younger age at onset, shorter survival, higher rates of cognitive and behavioral impairment, and a strong family history of neurodegeneration.

TDP-43, the pathological product of TARDBP, is present in pathological aggregates in almost all forms of FALS and SALS, and also in a subset of patients with FTD. TARDBP and FUS are involved in RNA processing, which has become an active field of research in ALS pathogenesis. These genes are not analyzed routinely in SALS patients. Rarely, mutations are identified.

Prognosis and treatment of ALS

Without treatment (Table 1.4), 50% of patients die within three years of onset; 10% of patients survive

Table 1.4. Treatment strategies in amyotrophic lateral sclerosis

Survival	
• Anti-glutamate drug riluzole	Prolongs survival by three months
• Noninvasive ventilation (NIV), if VC <50%, or if orthopnea is present	Prolongs survival in spinal-onset ALS by three months, may increase quality of life Not effective in severe bulbar ALS
• Multidisciplinary care	Prolongs survival and increases quality of life
• Vitamin E (antioxidant), creatine monohydrate, minocycline	Not effective
Weight loss	PEG: stabilizes body weight and may prolong life. Insufficient evidence to suggest specific timing of PEG insertion in ALS
Sialorrhea	Amitriptyline, scopolamine, glycopyrrolate, botulin toxin B, radiation therapy
Choking, thick mucus	N-acetylcysteine, propranolol, air stacking
Pseudobulbar signs	Amitriptyline, fluvoxamine, lithium carbonate, levodopa, or combined dextromethorphan and quinidine
Muscle cramps	Try carbamazepine or phenytoin
Spasticity	Mild training. Uncertain effect of spasmolytic drugs baclofen, dantrolene, and tizanidine
Musculoskeletal pain (immobilized patients)	Physical therapy and nonsteroidal anti-inflammatory drugs (NSAIDs)
Depression	Selective serotonin reuptake inhibitor (SSRI) or amitriptyline

beyond five years, and about 5% may survive for 10 years or more. Factors associated with a more rapid disease course are: shorter time to referral, age >50 years, bulbar onset, and rapid deterioration of pulmonary function. Management of patients in multidisciplinary clinics may prolong survival and enhance quality of life. This can be explained by experienced caregivers and by better adherence to practice parameters and diagnostic and treatment protocols. Comprehensive care is provided by dedicated and well-trained professionals including physicians, physical therapists, occupational and speech therapists, dieticians, social workers, and nurses. The team should collaborate closely with the GP and a center for respiratory support.

Great care must be taken when telling the patient that ALS is a fatal and progressive disease. Most patients will turn to the internet, which can be a shocking experience. We advocate a frank and open information strategy during all stages of the disease.

Most patients die either at home or in a hospice. Increasing hypercapnia causes gradual loss of consciousness. If dyspnoeic, morphine can alleviate symptoms. At this stage, anxiety can be treated with a benzodiazepine. A large number of patients die following continuous deep sedation. If the legal system and cultural circumstances permit, about one-fifth of patients with ALS decide on end-of-life practices– euthanasia and physician-assisted suicide, a higher proportion than in other life-threatening chronic diseases. This fact has not been associated with quality of care or depression.

Suggested reading

Andersen PM, Al-Chalabi A. Clinical genetics of amyotrophic lateral sclerosis: what do we really know? *Nat Rev Neurol* 2011; 7: 603–615.

Brooks B, Miller R, Swash M, Munsat T. El Escorial revisited: revised criteria for the diagnosis of amyotrophic lateral sclerosis. *Amyotroph Lateral Scler Other Motor Neuron Disord* 2000; 1: 293–299.

Byrne S, Elamin N, Bede P, et al. Cognitive and clinical characteristics of patients with amyotrophic lateral sclerosis carrying a C9 or f72 repeat expansion: a population-based cohort study. *Lancet Neurol* 2012; 11: 232–240.

Chiò A, Calvo A, Moglia C. Phenotypic heterogeneity of amyotrophic lateral sclerosis: a population based study. *J Neurol Neurosurg Psychiatry* 2011; 82: 740–746.

Dion PA, Daoud H, Rouleau GA. Genetics of motor neuron disorders: new insights into pathogeneic mechanisms. *Nature Rev Genet* 2009; 10: 769–782.

Huisman MH, De Jong SW, Van Doormaal PT, et al. Population based epidemiology of amyotrophic lateral sclerosis using capture-recapture methodology. *J Neurol Neurosurg Psychiatry* 2011; 82: 1165–1170.

Kiernan MC, Vusic S, Cheah BC, et al. Amyotrophic lateral sclerosis. *Lancet* 2011; 377: 942–955.

Logroscino G, Traynor BJ, Hardiman O, et al. Incidence of amyotrophic lateral sclerosis in Europe. *J Neurol Neurosurg Psychiatry* 2010; 81: 385–390.

Maessen M, Veldink J, Onwuteaka-Philipsen B, et al. Trends and determinants of end-of-life practices in ALS in the Netherlands. *Neurology* 2009; 73: 954–961.

Miller RG, Jackson CE, Kasarkis EJ, et al. Practice parameter update: the care of the patient with amyotrophic lateral sclerosis: drug, nutritional, and respiratory therapies (an evidence-based review). *Neurology* 2009: 73: 1218–1226.

Miller RG, Jackson CE, Kasarkis EJ, et al. Practice parameter update: the care of the patient with amyotrophic lateral sclerosis: multidisciplinary care, symptom management, and cognitive/behavioural impairment (an evidence-based review). *Neurology* 2009; 73: 1227–1233.

Renton AE, Majounie E, Waite A, et al. A hexanucleotide repeat expansion in C9ORF72 is the cause of chromosome 9p21-linked ALS–FTD. *Neuron* 2011; 20: 257–268.

Smith B, Newhouse S, Shatunov A, et al. The C9ORF72 expansion mutation is a common cause of ALS +/– FTD in Europe and has a single founder. Eur J Hum Genet 2012 [Epub ahead of print].

Sutedja NA, Veldink J, Fischer K, et al. Lifetime occupation, education, smoking and risk of ALS. *Neurology* 2007; 9: 508–514.

Traynor BJ, Codd MB, Corr B, et al. Clinical features of amyotrophic lateral sclerosis according to the El Escorial and Airlie House diagnostic criteria. A population-based study. *Arch Neurol* 2000; 57: 1171–1176.

Van der Graaff MC, Grolman W, Westermann EJ, et al. Vocal cord dysfunction in amyotrophic lateral sclerosis: four cases and a review of the literature. *Arch Neurol* 2009; 66: 1329–1333.

www.wfnals.org

Amyotrophic lateral sclerosis with frontotemporal dementia: an engineer who laughed too loudly

Clinical history

For about six months, a 49-year-old engineer had increasing difficulties with fastening buttons, knotting his tie, and handling a drill. For the past year, he had noticed twitches in muscles of both arms. He had no other symptoms.

Cautiously, his wife mentioned behavioral changes. Onset was about two years before onset of his motor problems, when he had a burn-out. He never fully recovered. He was easily irritated and could react with emotional outbursts. At times, he made inappropriate and embarrassing remarks.

She knew him as an introvert person, but for about a year he had been laughing more loudly than his eight-year-old son when watching cartoons on television. He had difficulties executing tasks; for example emptying the dishwasher. The family history was negative.

Examination

He was apathetic and did not show much emotion. He was fully oriented with a normal Mini-Mental State Examination (MMSE). He had no overt dysphasia, but had difficulty explaining proverbs. He could not spell backwards. He could not easily name series of objects. He showed perseverance when performing several tasks.

The tongue showed fasciculations and decrease of rapid movements. He had atrophic muscles in the right hand and vivid fasciculation of proximal muscles of arms and legs. Muscles of both shoulders and arms were weakened, more so on the right side and more distally. Abdominal skin reflexes were absent and he had a left Babinski sign. He could not rise easily from a chair and had an asymmetric, spastic gait.

Ancillary investigations

The EMG showed LMN signs in the cervical, thoracic, and lumbosacral regions. VC was 104%. An MRI scan of the brain showed atrophy, especially frontotemporal.

Diagnostic considerations

He was diagnosed with ALS and cognitive decline suggestive of FTD.

Follow-up

He was treated with riluzole, 50 mg twice daily. After three months, behavioral changes became more evident and weakness of both arms increased. VC had decreased to 91% and he experienced weight loss. He had to be admitted to a nursing home where he died 18 months after onset of hand weakness.

General remarks

Mild cognitive impairment with subtle performance deficits occurs in many ALS patients. A minority of patients has the frontal, behavioral variant of FTD. Alternatively, ALS may develop in patients with FTD. Semantic dementia and progressive nonfluent aphasia, other phenotypes of frontotemporal lobar degeneration, are much less prevalent. From a systematic review of the publications on behavioral changes in ALS, the prevalence of the behavioral variant of FTD has been estimated to be 8.1% (95% CI, 5.6%–11.5%). Until population-based data become available, the true incidence will remain unknown. Additionally, the natural history of cognitive decline and of FTD in ALS has not been studied systematically. A continuum between mild cognitive impairment and overt FTD seems unlikely. The repeat expansion in the C9ORF72 hexanucleotide gene has a characteristic phenotype with younger age at onset, shorter survival, higher rates of cognitive and behavioral impairment, and a strong family history of neurodegeneration (see Case 1).

Symptoms of FTD in ALS include personality change, irritability, poor insight, disinhibition, perseveration, apathy, and severe performance deficits. Progressive deterioration of FTD has been observed in many patients with ALS.

Neuropathological and genetic studies have demonstrated that ALS–FTD forms a heterogeneous complex of diseases. The clinician must be aware that cognitive and behavioral changes form part of the spectrum of ALS, especially in the bulbar-onset form. The story of the partner or a family member can lead to the diagnosis. The MMSE cannot be used for screening for FTD. The frontal assessment battery may prove a promising method of screening for frontal lobe dysfunction in ALS, but many patients have motor impairment that make testing impossible. Patients with impaired verbal fluency probably have deficits in frontal executive

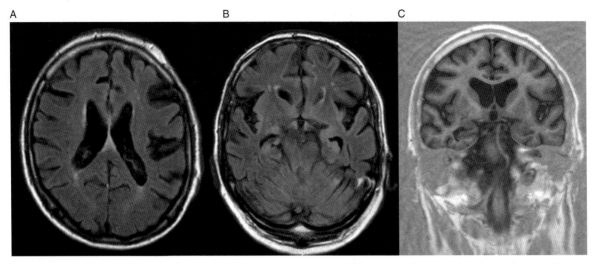

Figure 2.1. ALS and behavioral variant frontotemporal dementia. Man, 71 years old. Progressive dyspnea and weakness of arms and legs, cognitive decline and inappropriate social behavior, and urinary and fecal incontinence. VC 43% of expected, weakness in the cervical, thoracic, and lumbosacral regions with hyperreflexia of the arms. MRI of the brain ([A, B] FLAIR; [C] T1-weighted images): cortical atrophy in the frontal and temporal areas with hippocampal atrophy.

function. Localized cortical atrophy can be observed in ALS–FTD (Figure 2.1).

The clinical implications are important. Difficulties with attention span, planning, and judgment can have negative consequences for patient care as there will be a greater degree of noncompliance with PEG and NIV. Patients with performance dysfunction have a shorter survival time. As social conduct can alter and emotions are increasingly not recognized by patients, special attention must be paid to partners and caregivers.

Suggested reading

Elamin M, Phukan J, Bede P, et al. Executive dysfunction is a negative prognostic indicator in patients with ALS without dementia. *Neurology* 2011; **76**: 1262–1269.

Miller RG, Jackson CE, Kasarskis EJ. Practice parameter update: the care of the patient with amyotrophic lateral sclerosis: multidisciplinary care, symptom management, and cognitive/behavioral impairment (an evidence-based review). *Neurology* 2009; **73**: 1227–1233.

Neary D, Snowden JS, Gustafson L, et al. Frontotemporal lobe degeneration: a consensus on diagnostic criteria. *Neurology* 1998; **51**: 1546–1554.

Phukan J, Pender NP, Hardiman O. Cognitive impairment in amyotrophic lateral sclerosis. *Lancet Neurol* 2007; **6**: 994–1003.

Raaphorst J, Beeldman E, De Visser M, De Haan RJ, Schmand B. A systematic review of behavioural changes in motor neuron disease. *Amyotroph Lateral Scler* 2012; **13**: 493–501.

Primary lateral sclerosis: a cobbler who could no longer play tennis

Case history

At about the age of 40 years, a male cobbler, now 53 years old, noted difficulty playing tennis. He could no longer switch easily from one leg to another and missed the ball at the net. Serving went well. After a game, he noted pain in both legs. At 43 years old, he stopped taking part in competitions, and five years later had to give up playing altogether. At that time, he sometimes missed the brake and accelerator pedals of his car. Walking became increasingly difficult. Sometimes he nearly fell due to weakness of his left leg and he had to use a walking stick. From the age of 50 years, he used a wheelchair to go outside. At 52 years old, he could only work part-time as his dexterity decreased. Urinary continence was not a problem, but when he felt the urge, he had to rush to the toilet. His family history was not informative.

Examination

He had a snout reflex and a hyperactive masseter reflex. His arm reflexes were brisk. Muscle tone of both legs was increased and he had mild weakness of hip and knee flexor and foot extensor muscles. His knee reflexes showed a clonus and he had Babinski signs. He had a spastic gait that increased with distance.

Ancillary investigations

Previous analysis had shown no vitamin B12 deficiency, normal cerebrospinal fluid (CSF) and normal MRI scans of the spine and head. The EMG was normal. Normal serum (very) long-chain fatty acid ratios excluded adrenomyeloneuropathy. Mutation analysis for hereditary spastic paresis was negative.

Diagnostic considerations

The slowly progressive spastic syndrome without LMN signs and normal test results led to a diagnosis of PLS.

Follow-up

We could reassure the patient that the odds of not developing ALS were extremely high and, second, that his life expectancy was estimated to be normal. He did, however, have to take account of the fact that his action radius would decrease further and that manual dexterity could become a problem over the years.

General remarks

PLS is a diagnosis by exclusion (Table 3.1) that has been redefined as part of the spectrum of ALS/MND (see Case 1, Figure 1.2). By definition, PLS is a sporadic disease without abnormalities on extensive ancillary investigations, and a suggested follow-up period of at least three years with no alternative diagnosis. Patients with rapid progression may evolve to ALS.

In our series, median age at onset was 49 years (range 18–76 yr). About 87% of patients had onset in the leg. Onset in the bulbar or arm regions was less frequent (Video 6). Asymmetric onset was reported in half of the patients, asymmetry on examination in one of five cases. Strict unilateral signs were rare. About 40% of patients had urinary urgency. Decreased vibratory sense and focal amyotrophy occurred in 9% of cases. After a median disease duration of six years, 43% of patients had pure leg involvement, 17% had involvement of legs and arms, and 40% had bulbar signs. There is substantial overlap of phenotypes between PLS and hereditary spastic paraplegia (HSP) with mutations in SPG4, SPG7, and possibly other yet unrecognized genes. Current clinical criteria are not always useful for distinguishing between PLS and HSP in individual patients.

BSCL2 or seipin gene mutations cause variants of CMT2 disease (see Case 11), distal hereditary upper limb motor neuropathy type V, Silver syndrome–amyotrophy of the hand muscles and spasticity of the lower limbs, and HSP17 (Figure 3.1).

Suggested reading

Brugman F, Veldink JH, Franssen H, et al. Differentiation of hereditary spastic paresis from primary lateral sclerosis in psoradic adult-onset upper motor neuron syndromes. *Arch Neurol* 2009; **66**: 509–514.

Irobi J, Van den Bergh P, Merlini L, et al. The phenotype of motor neuropathies associated with BSCL2 mutations is broader than Silver syndrome land distal HMN type V. *Brain* 2004; **127**: 2124–2130.

Table 3.1. Causes of adult-onset chronic progressive spastic paraplegia

Disease	Characteristic features
Primary progressive MS	1-year disease progression 2 out of: positive brain MRI/positive spinal cord MRI/positive CSF (high IgG-index, oligoclonals bands) No other explanation
Cervical spondylarthrotic myelopathy	Sensory symptoms may occur in hands Cervical stenosis with myelopathy on MRI (Video 12)
Other structural lesions: intra-axial or extra-axial spinal tumor Calcified herniated thoracic disk Arnold–Chiari malformation Os odontoideum Rheumatoid arthritis of the upper cervical spine	MRI shows characteristic abnormalities Cervical lesions may have false signs suggesting abnormality at thoracic level
Vitamin B12 deficiency	Usually prominent dysfunction of proprioception Abnormal full blood cyanocobalamin (B12), fasting plasma homocysteine, plasma methylmalonic acid MRI may show dorsal myelopathy
Human T-cell lymphocytotropic virus type 1 (HTLV1) infection (tropic spastic paraparesis)	Years after infection with HTLV1, patients may develop chronic spastic paraparesis. Endemic areas have been detected in the Caribbean, South America, sub-Saharan Africa, and Japan. Patients may have associated neuropathy
Neurosarcoidosis	High serum and CSF angiotensin-converting enzyme (ACE) (not obligatory) High CSF IgG-index and oligoclonal banding MRI of spinal cord shows myelopathy
Krabbe disease	Brain MRI shows lesions in internal capsules Low plasma galactocerebrosidase activity
Adrenomyeloneuropathy	Usually prominent dysfunction of proprioception Abnormal serum very long-chain fatty acid ratios DNA analysis of the ABCD1 gene
Pure HSP	DNA analysis of AD SPG4 (40% of adult HSP), AD SPG 3A (10%), AD SPG 7 (sometimes with cerebellar ataxia), and other SPG genes
Copper deficiency myelopathy	Treatable-cause myelopathy mimicking subacute combined degeneration due to vitamin B12 deficiency. Risk factors are previous upper gastrointestinal surgery and zinc overload
PLS	Diagnosis by exclusion

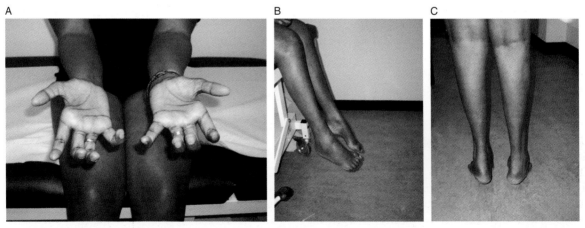

A B C

Figure 3.1. A 46-year-old woman with Silver syndrome caused by a BSCL2 gene mutation. Atrophy of lower leg muscles started at the age of eight years, with the hands becoming involved later. She had gradual progression of walking difficulties. On examination, she had claw hands with severe distal muscle atrophy and weakness (A), and bilateral pes equinovarus and atrophy of lower leg muscles (B). She could not put her heels to the ground (C). Clonus of the knee reflexes, absent Achilles jerks and bilateral Babinski signs were noted.

Jaiser SR, Winston GP. Copper deficiency myelopathy. *J Neurol* 2010; **257**: 869–881.

Polman CH, Reingold SC, Banwell B, et al. Diagnostic criteria for multiple sclerosis: 2010 revisions to the McDonald criteria. *Ann Neurol* 2011; **69**: 292–302.

Verdonck K, González E, Van Dooren S, et al. Human T-lymphocytotropic virus 1: recent knowledge about an ancient infection. *Lancet Infect Dis* 2007; 7: 266–281.

Younger DS, Chou S, Hays AP, et al. Primary lateral sclerosis: a clinical diagnosis reemerges. *Arch Neurol* 1988; **45**: 1304–1307.

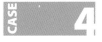

Progressive muscular atrophy: an accordionist with cramps in one arm

Clinical history

When playing slow passages, a 55-year-old professional accordionist noticed painless cramps of the finger flexor muscles of the right hand. Treatment with botulin toxin for suspected dystonia had no effect. In the following months cramps also occurred when at rest and he had to give up his profession. He noted twitches in the limb muscles.

Examination

On inspection, he had widespread fasciculations in the shoulder, chest, and abdominal wall muscles. There was no skeletal muscle atrophy and no weakness. Muscle tendon reflexes were normal and there were no Babinski signs.

Ancillary investigations

CK activity was at the upper limit of normal. EMG revealed fasciculation potentials in the deltoid, biceps brachii, dorsal interosseus, rectus femoris, and anterior tibial muscles but no spontaneous muscle fiber activity, possibly indicating denervation. Nerve conduction studies were normal. There were no conduction blocks. An MRI scan of the neck offered no explanation.

Follow-up

Two years after diagnosis, he experienced more fasciculation and difficulties turning a key and clipping his nails. Three years after onset, dexterity of the arms decreased. He had weakness of the extensor muscles of both wrists and fingers. At that time, EMG showed spontaneous muscle fiber activity and neurogenic MUPs, suggesting an ongoing process of denervation and reinnervation. He was diagnosed with progressive muscular atrophy (PMA).

Four years after diagnosis, walking became difficult. Expected forced VC decreased from 53% to 39%. With NIV, day-time fatigue and sleepiness improved. Nine years after diagnosis, he developed tongue atrophy, weakness, and dysphagia. At that time, distal limb muscles were paralytic with some proximal strength preserved. Shortly afterward he died. Pyramidal signs were never observed.

General remarks

Since PMA was first described by Aran in 1850, the possible existence of a nosological entity distinct from ALS has been considered. Corticospinal tract degeneration in the spinal cord and brainstem has been demonstrated in patients with PMA. Additionally, during the disease course, a fair proportion of patients with PMA develop pyramidal features.

PMA may evolve from segmental muscular atrophy that is characterized by weakness and atrophy restricted to one or two limbs, usually the arms. Involvement of one arm may lead to a flail arm syndrome. With both arms, a "man-in-the-barrel" syndrome can occur (Figure 4.1). Atrophy and weakness of paraspinal and truncal muscles causes head drop, shoulder drooping, or stooped posture. Progressive bulbar palsy is an uncommon bulbar-onset LMN syndrome.

In a recent, prospective, population-based study of clinical features in 388 Irish patients, 8% had suspected ALS at onset and only 2% after six years. This suggests that many patients with PMA develop UMN signs and thus ALS. All patients with PMA show relentless progression. Median survival after initial weakness is about five years, compared with three years in ALS. Rapidly decreasing VC is associated with poor prognosis.

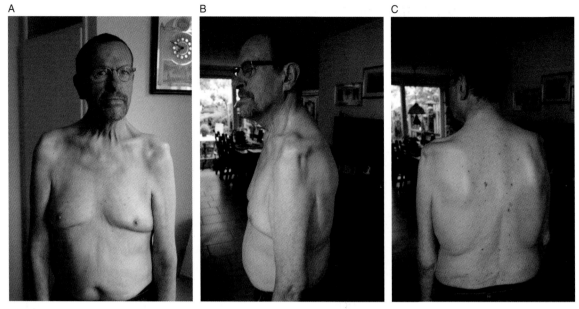

Figure 4.1. (A–C) Man-in-the-barrel or flail arm syndrome. The patient shown could no longer use the atrophic and weak muscles of both shoulders and upper arms. He retained some grip function of the hands.

Due to the rarity of the condition, it is not known whether the anti-glutamate drug, riluzole, is also effective in PMA. It is common practice to prescribe riluzole to PMA patients. In addition, rehabilitation medicine has a large role. NIV is indicated in patients with orthopnea or a forced VC below 50% (see Case 1).

Suggested reading

Ince PG, Evans J, Knopp M, et al. Corticospinal tract degeneration in the progressive muscular atrophy variant of ALS. *Neurology* 2003; **60**: 1252–1258.

Traynor BJ, Codd MB, Corr B, et al. Clinical features of amyotrophic lateral sclerosis according to the El Escorial and Airlie House diagnostic criteria. A population-based study. *Arch Neurol* 2000; **57**: 1171–1176.

Van den Berg-Vos RM, Visser J, Franssen H, et al. Sporadic lower motor neuron disease with adult onset: classification of subtypes. *Brain* 2003; **126**: 1036–1047.

Visser J, van den Berg-Vos RM, Franssen H. Disease course and prognostic factors of progressive muscular atrophy. *Arch Neurol* 2007; **64**: 522–528.

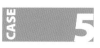

Kennedy disease: a man with swimming difficulties, who was insecure at night

Clinical history

A 58-year-old man had to give up his weekly swimming club as, gradually, he could no longer keep up with his peers and had difficulty climbing out of the water. He had always been a keen hiker, but for the past four years had to shorten the distance. His body weight increased. Six months ago, he sprained his ankle after stumbling over a threshold and falling. In the dark, he had to take great care to find his way and not to fall. He tended to choke when drinking a cup of hot tea. Ten years ago, he had been treated for pulmonary sarcoidosis with prednisone. His mother's deceased brother, who had been a postman, had become wheelchair-dependent after retiring.

Examination

He was obese with a BMI of 40. No gynecomastia was observed. He had perioral fasciculations, most obvious in the mentalis muscle (Video 10). The edges of his tongue were serrated with fasciculations. The strength of his tongue and facial muscles appeared normal. He had a postural and kinetic tremor of both arms (Video 10). He had a limb girdle pattern of weakness with affected deltoid, supraspinatus, infraspinatus, and iliopsoas muscles (Video 10). Pain sense was normal, but vibration sense was decreased below the knees. The Achilles tendon reflexes were absent.

Ancillary investigations

CK activity was six times ULN. EMG showed sporadic spontaneous muscle fiber activity and long-duration, giant MUPs, suggesting denervation and collateral sprouting, in various muscles of the face and limbs. All sensory nerve action potential amplitudes were decreased. The appropriate DNA test revealed 51 CAG-repeats in the androgen receptor gene (normal <40).

Diagnostic considerations

The combination of adult-onset limb girdle syndrome in males, perioral fasciculation, sensory neuropathy, and positive family history with affected males suggests a diagnosis of Kennedy disease, spinal and bulbar muscular atrophy.

Follow-up

VC was 69% of expected and decreased over three years. He received NIV. Weakness gradually progressed but he remained ambulatory.

General remarks

Kennedy disease is caused by CAG trinucleotide repeat expansion (range 40–62 repeats) in exon 1 of the androgen receptor gene on the X-chromosome, the consequent polyglutamine expanded androgen receptor aggregates in nuclei of motor neurons and dorsal root ganglion cells causing neuronal dysfunction and ultimate loss. In essence, Kennedy disease is a neuronopathy and not a length-dependent axonopathy. The size of the repeat expansion correlates negatively with age at onset.

Within affected families, the phenotype may vary (Table 5.1). As Kennedy disease progresses slowly over the years, the description of the phenotype depends on the duration of the symptomatic phase. Symptoms and signs that may precede weakness include CK elevation, muscle cramps and myalgia in up to 50% of cases, easy fatigue, and postural tremor of the hands. The average delay from onset of weakness to diagnosis has been calculated to be more than five years. There is an inverse relationship between CAG repeat length and age at diagnosis and muscle strength. Endocrinological abnormalities, such as reduced fertility and gynecomastia, form part of the clinical spectrum. Female carriers can experience muscle cramps in the calves at night, mildly elevated CK activity, and a neurogenic EMG.

Prevalence of Kennedy disease in the male population has been estimated to be 3:100 000. Progression is slow and life expectancy is near normal.

Suggested reading

Finsterer J. Perspectives of Kennedy disease. *J Neurol Sci* 2010; **298**: 1–10.

Lee J-H, Shin J-H, Park K-P, et al. Phenotypic variability in Kennedy's disease: implication of the early diagnostic features. *Acta Neurol Scand* 2005; **112**: 57–63.

Rhodes LE, Freeman BK, Auh S, et al. Clinical features of spinal and bulbar muscular atrophy. *Brain* 2009; **132**: 3242–3251.

Table 5.1. Phenotype of Kennedy disease at evaluation

Age at onset (yr)	Fifth decade. Onset can be in early 20s and after 65
Mean time to diagnosis	>10 (yr)
Weakness	Usually limb girdle pattern, sometimes bulbar or hand onset. Asymmetry can occur
Bulbar symptoms	Mild dysarthria (nasal voice), slight dysphagia, perioral and tongue fasciculation, weak facial muscles, jaw drop
Premature exhaustion	>80%
Muscle cramps, myalgia	>50%, mostly exercise-induced
Postural and kinetic tremor	90% (7–10 Hz), voice tremor >60%
Sensory impairment	>40% (distal loss of pain and vibration sense)
Gynecomastia[a]	>50%
CK elevation	1.5–15 x ULN

[a] Gynecomastia: undurated mass under the nipple or enlarged mammary gland mass.

Sperfeld AD, Karitzky J, Brummer D, et al. X-linked bulbopsinal neuronopathy. Kennedy disease. *Arch Neurol* 2002; **59**: 1921–1926.

Suzuki K, Katsuno M, Banno H, et al. CAG repeat size correlates to motor and sensory phenotypes in SBMA. *Brain* 2008; **131**: 229–239.

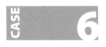

CASE 6

Spinal muscular atrophy type 3, Kugelberg–Welander disease: two sisters who could no longer climb stairs

Clinical history

Patient A, a 20-year-old courier, was examined because of frequent falls due to weakness of the legs. From the age of 12, she could not keep up with her peers at sport. Many years of physical therapy had no effect. She had no complaints when cycling. After 20 minutes' walking, she complained of pain and weakness in the legs. At the time of referral, she had problems rising from a sitting position. She did not have cramps.

Patient B, her 15-year-old sister, had no spontaneous complaints. After climbing a third flight of stairs, she experienced difficulty raising her legs. After running to catch a bus, she developed cramp in the hamstring muscles.

Examination

Patient A had no muscle atrophy. She had symmetric weakness of the shoulder abductor, hip abductor, and knee extensor muscles, MRC grade 4–5, and hip abductor muscles, MRC grade 4. Weakness of the knee flexor muscles was asymmetric: MRC grade 4 on the right side and MRC grade 3 on the left side. The knee reflexes were absent. Sensation was normal. There were no joint contractures or scoliosis. She had a positive Gowers' sign and a waddling gait.

Patient B had normal results on MMT. The knee reflexes were absent. When rising from a squatting position she had to keep her balance by placing one leg forward.

There was no fasciculation.

Ancillary investigations

Elevation of serum CK activity was mild in both cases (<2 × ULN). EMG did not show denervation activity. In patient A, a CT scan of the muscular system showed widespread atrophy of muscles of both legs. A skeletal muscle biopsy revealed larged group atrophy and type grouping of muscle fibers (Figure 6.1).

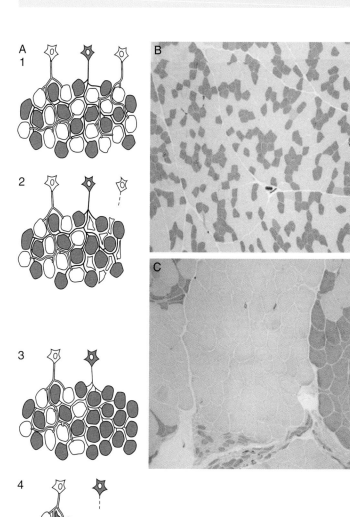

Figure 6.1. (A) Schematic drawing of the process of denervation and reinnervation: (1) normal checkerboard pattern of type 1 and type 2 muscle fibers; (2) atrophy following denervation as one motor neuron cell degenerates; (3) reinnervation of most atrophied muscle fibers by new nerve endings (sprouts) from the axon of a nearby motor neuron cell. A group of muscle fibers of the same type is formed, "type grouping," with loss of the checkerboard pattern; (4) atrophy of all muscle fibers belonging to that group of muscle fibers as the second motor neuron cell degenerates, "grouped atrophy." (B) Checkerboard pattern of type 1 and type 2 muscle fibers. (C) Type-grouping and grouped atrophy (muscle biopsy section stained with ATPase, pH 4.3, staining type 1 fibers dark and type 2 fibers light).

Diagnostic considerations

The gradual onset of a limb girdle syndrome before the age of 30 years in two family members associated with chronic neurogenic abnormalities in the muscle biopsy led to a diagnosis of hereditary spinal muscular atrophy (SMA) type 3. Mutation analysis of the SMN1 gene was requested.

Follow-up

In both girls, homozygous deletions of exons 7 and 8 of the SMN1 gene confirmed a diagnosis of late-onset SMA type 3, or Kugelberg–Welander disease.

During a three-year follow-up, they complained of increasing fatigue and weakness, but MMT results

using the MRC scale did not change. VC remained normal. The other four siblings from this family all proved to be carriers of the same mutations in the SMN1 genes. In addition, all had four copies of the SMN2 gene. During follow-up, two younger brothers aged 12 and 16 years reported a postural tremor of the hands, which can be a first sign of SMA. Genetic testing showed that they also had late-onset SMA type 3.

General remarks

SMA is among the neuromuscular disorders that are the leading genetic cause of infant death. Age at onset and age at reaching motor milestones (i.e., sitting and walking) define subtypes of SMA (Table 6.1). SMA is

Table 6.1. Phenotypes of survival motor neuron gene-related spinal muscular atrophy

	SMA1 Werdnig–Hoffmann disease	SMA2 Intermediate type	SMA3 Kugelberg–Welander disease	SMA4 Adult-onset (very rare)
Age at onset	Antenatal–before 6 mo	7–18 mo	After 18 mo–30 yr	After 30 yr
Maximum motor milestones	Never sits independently	Sits independently Never walks independently	Walks independently Some patients become wheelchair-dependent in childhood	Normal
Other features	Floppy child, no control of head movements, normal facial expression, swallowing difficulty; paradoxal breathing Fasciculation of the tongue	Scoliosis, joint contractures Postural tremors of the hands Fasciculations of tongue and/or limb muscles	Scoliosis, joint contractures Postural tremors of the hands Fasciculations of limb muscles Some patients require NIV (monitor VC every year)	Patients can become wheelchair-dependent Some patients require NIV (monitor VC every year)
Life expectancy	Median survival <6 mo Death from respiratory insufficiency	Most patients die <age 30–40 yr from respiratory insufficiency, some survive longer	Normal	Normal

Classification of SMA is being made on the basis of age at onset and of achieved motor milestones. Patients with early onset SMA type 3a have been able to walk independently, but experience manifestations of SMA before the age of three years. In one study, probability of being ambulatory at age 20 years was much lower compared with patients with SMA type 3b who had first manifestations after the age of three years (44% vs. 89%).

caused by degeneration of motor neuron cells in the lower brainstem and spinal cord. Neurons of extraocular muscles and facial muscles are spared. Swallowing is affected, especially in the early childhood forms. SMA type 1, Werdnig–Hoffmann disease, is the most severe and frequent phenotype.

Prospective natural history studies of late-onset SMA type 3 and SMA type 4 patients show a fairly uniform phenotype with leg-onset limb girdle weakness and slow progression. Fatigue is an early complaint in most patients. In the course of the disease, some patients lose the ability to walk unaided; few need a wheelchair.

Inheritance is autosomal recessive (AR). The incidence is about 1:10 000 live births with a carrier frequency of 1 in 50. Over 95% of SMA patients have homozygous deletions of exons 7 and 8 of the SMN genes. Interestingly, similar deletions have been reported in unaffected or only mildly affected siblings of patients with SMA type 3. These findings suggest a role for modifier genes. Chromosome 5 has one telomeric SMN1 gene and one or more copies of the centromeric SMN2 gene on chromosome 5q13. The SMN2 gene differs only slightly from the SMN1 gene, but only about 10% of the gene product of the SMN2 gene is translated into full-length SMN protein. Phenotypic differences can be explained partially by the number of SMN2 gene copies as a higher number of correlates with a milder phenotype. Patient A and patient B had four copies. Five per cent of patients have a type of SMN1 gene mutation other than deletions of exons 7 and 8. Most of these are compound heterozygotes with a deletion of one SMN1 allele and a point mutation or other small mutations in the other allele.

Diagnostic tips on how to recognize late-onset SMA type 3 and SMA type 4 cases are presented in Table 6.2. Late-onset SMA type 3 and SMA type 4 patients may develop joint contractures and become wheelchair-dependent. Physical therapy is indicated to treat pain that results from inactivity and contractures. Pulmonary function must be monitored at regular intervals. NIV may be indicated.

Table 6.2. Diagnostic tips for recognition of patients with late-onset spinal muscular atrophy types 3 and 4

- More or less symmetric limb girdle syndrome with slow progression over months–years, or indiscriminate weakness associated with fasciculation and polyminimyoclonus

- CK normal–slightly elevated (<10 x ULN)

- EMG: pattern of denervation and reinnervation, normal motor and sensory conduction. Note: a normal EMG does not exclude a diagnosis of SMA

- If EMG suggests neurogenic abnormalities, screen for a mutation in the SMN1 gene

- If EMG is normal, consider a skeletal muscle biopsy. If compatible with a neurogenic cause, screen for a mutation in the SMN1 gene

- If no mutation is found, reconsider the diagnosis. Consider whether extensive analysis of nerve conduction is indicated to exclude CIDP (Case 16). Some CIDP cases have very slow progression and only proximal conduction abnormalities that can be hard to find

- Store DNA for future screening of other not yet identified genes

Suggested reading

Bussaglia E, Tizzano EF, Illa I. et al. Cramps and minimal EMG abnormalities as preclinical manifestations of spinal muscular atrophy patients with homozygous deletions of the SMN gene. *Neurology* 1997; **48**: 1443–1445.

Cobben JM, van der Steege G, Grootscholten P, et al. Deletions of the survival motor neuron gene in unaffected siblings of patients with spinal muscular atrophy. *Am J Hum Genet* 1995; **57**: 805–808.

Lunn MR, Wang CH. Spinal muscular atrophy. *Lancet* 2008; **371**: 2120–2133.

Piepers S, van den Berg LH, Brugman F, et al. A natural history study of late onset spinal muscular atrophy types 3 and b. *J Neurol* 2008; **255**: 1400–1404.

Prior TW. Spinal muscular atrophy diagnostics. *J Child Neurol* 2007; **22**: 952–956.

Zerres K, Rudnik-Schöneborn S, Forrest E, et al. A collaborative study on the natural history of childhood and juvenile onset proximal spinal muscular atrophy (type II and III SMA): 569 patients. *J Neurol Sci* 1997; **147**: 67–72.

Zerres K, Rudnik-Schöneborn S. Natural history in proximal spinal muscular attrophy. Clinical analysis of 445 patients and suggestions for a modification of existing classifications. *Arch Neurol* 1995; **52**: 518–523.

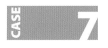

CASE 7

Postpoliomyelitis syndrome: a retired psychoanalyst who was misdiagnosed as spinal muscular atrophy type 3

Clinical history

In 1956, the patient, who at that time was 18 years old, experienced onset of weakness in his left arm and both legs associated with a fever. No diagnosis was reached. He gradually recovered but had residual weakness of the pelvic girdle muscles, which made it difficult for him to get up from a chair. In 1958, a diagnosis of spinal muscular atrophy (SMA) type 3 was made.

He remained stable during adulthood. Following a patellar fracture after a fall at age 61 years, he noticed a gradual decrease in strength of the leg muscles, more pronounced in the right leg. At the age of 73 years, he was reassessed because the (referring) neurologist considered a postpolio syndrome to be more likely, thus refuting the previous diagnosis of SMA type 3.

Examination

He had atrophy of the muscles of his upper legs and a positive Gowers' sign. Achilles tendon jerks were negative, but no other abnormalities were found.

Ancillary investigations

A skeletal CT scan showed replacement of the right quadriceps femoris muscle by adipose tissue with some fatty infiltration in the left quadriceps muscle (Figure 7.1).

Diagnostic considerations

A diagnosis of SMA type 3, Kugelberg–Welander syndrome, was unlikely (Case 6), as initially the patient

Table 7.1. Criteria for postpoliomyelitis syndrome

1. Prior paralytic poliomyelitis with evidence of motor neuron loss, as confirmed by a history of the acute paralytic illness, signs of residual weakness, and atrophy of muscles on neurological examination, or signs of denervation on EMG

2. Period of partial or complete functional recovery after acute paralytic poliomyelitis, followed by an interval (≥15 yr) of stable neurological function

3. Gradual or sudden onset of progressive and persistent muscle weakness or abnormal fatigability (i.e., decreased endurance), with or without generalized fatigue, muscle atrophy, or muscle and joint pain. Sudden onset may follow a period of inactivity, trauma, or surgery. Less frequent symptoms attributed to PPS include new difficulties with swallowing or breathing

4. Symptoms and signs persisting for at least one year

5. No other neurological, orthopedic, or medical explanation

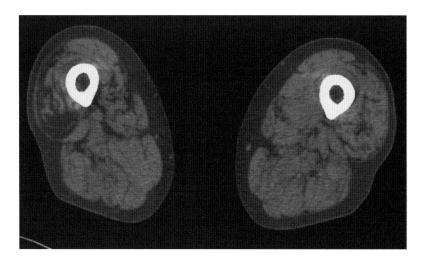

Figure 7.1. Both quadriceps femoris muscles show areas of lower attenuation, right more than left, in a patient with postpoliomyelitis syndrome, who complained about progressive gait difficulty.

experienced asymmetric muscle weakness associated with fever followed by gradual improvement in muscle strength, and subsequently, a stable phase lasting many years. It is highly likely that he had suffered from poliomyelitis anterior acuta. Because, after a period of stability, he complained of increased muscle weakness in the legs that had previously been affected, a diagnosis of postpoliomyelitis syndrome (PPS) was established.

General remarks

Several years after acute paralytic poliomyelitis, many poliomyelitis survivors experience new or increased muscle weakness, new atrophy, fatigue, muscular and joint pain, and cold intolerance. The term PPS was introduced by Halstead in 1985 (Table 7.1).

PPS has been reported in 15%–80% of all poliomyelitis survivors depending on the criteria applied and the population studied.

To reach a diagnosis, medical history taking and clinical examination usually suffice. If there is any doubt about a history of poliomyelitis, EMG may be helpful in demonstrating LMN involvement. Usually, signs of reinnervation prevail, spontaneous muscle fiber activity being minimal or absent. Imaging of the skeletal muscles is very useful as asymmetric involvement of limbs in which muscles are partially or completely replaced by fat indicate a past history of poliomyelitis.

It is of utmost importance to exclude other conditions that may mimic PPS. We have encountered patients who have had poliomyelitis and have residual sequelae and who developed other disorders such as syringomyelia (sensory abnormalities were the key feature here), muscle amyloidosis (rapid disease course), and entrapment neuropathies, especially in individuals using crutches.

The outcome of a systematic review of the effects of any treatment for PPS compared to placebo, usual care, or no treatment was that, because of insufficient good quality data and lack of randomized studies, it is impossible to draw definite conclusions about the effectiveness of interventions for PPS. Results indicate that IVIg, lamotrigine, muscle strengthening exercises, and static magnetic fields may be beneficial, but require further investigation.

Since the end of the twentieth century, poliomyelitis with acute flaccid paralysis caused by infection with West Nile virus (WNV), has been increasingly diagnosed in Africa, the Middle-East, and Japan. In 60%–80% of cases, WNV infections are asymptomatic. In <1%, there are neurological complications including meningitis, encephalitis, and poliomyelitis, or a combination of these. WNV–poliomyelitis typically manifests with asymmetric muscle weakness within 48 hours after the appearance of general signs of infection. Initially, there is a rapid increase of flaccid paresis, which may remain stable, or progress to tetraparesis, bulbar weakness, respiratory insufficiency, and

eventually death. The combination of the clinical picture, CSF pleocytosis, and detection of anti-WNV IgM antibodies in serum or CSF lead to a diagnosis. Polymerase chain reaction (PCR) of the serum does not have additional value as WNV-viremia is short-lived. WNV viral meningoencephalitis is now ubiquitous in North and Central America.

Suggested reading

Davis LE, De Biasi R, Goade DE, et al. West Nile virus neuroinvasive disease. *Ann Neurol* 2006; **60**: 286–300.

Farbu E, Gilhus NE, Barnes MP, et al. Post-polio syndrome. In: Gilhus NE, Brainin M, Barnes MP, eds. *European Handbook of Neurological Management*. Vol. 1. 2nd edn. Wiley–Blackwell, Oxford, 2011.

Koopman FS, Uegaki K, Gilhus NE, et al. Treatment for postpolio syndrome. *Cochrane Database Syst Rev* 2011; **2**: CD007818.

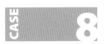

8 Spinal dural fistula: a train driver who had to curtail walking distances

Clinical history

A 67-year-old former train driver was referred for diagnosis of neuropathy. For two years he had experienced walking difficulties, which started with mild left-sided foot drop after walking some distance. His walking distance decreased, and due to weakness of the left leg, he could no longer reach the train station to train-spot. When walking and standing for some time, both legs felt like "pudding." This feeling decreased when bending forward. For five years, he had experienced spontaneous muscle cramps at the back of his left leg. During the past year, morning erections had disappeared. He had had colitis ulcerosa for 25 years, and severe varicosis of the legs for the past eight years.

Examination

He had mild atrophy of the left calf, weakness of the hip and knee flexors and of the hip and foot extensors, MRC grade 4. Trendelenburg sign was positive when standing on the left leg. In the prone position, knee flexion caused painful muscle cramps. Sensation was

normal. He had areflexia of the legs with a normal plantar response.

Ancillary investigations

Laboratory analysis of the blood was normal. EMG showed denervation activity in the leg and paraspinal muscles. Motor and sensory nerve conduction was normal. A spine T2-weighted MRI sequence revealed a large longitudinal hyperintense lesion in the spinal cord (Figure 8.1).

Diagnostic considerations

The clinical syndrome of increasing motor abnormalities in both legs with asymmetric onset, areflexia, and normal sensation could suggest slowly progressive PMA, the motor variant of CIDP, or myelopathy. EMG excluded CIDP. The MRI abnormalities are not a feature of PMA. These have been described in spinal dural arteriovenous fistula (SDAVF). Gait claudication is compatible with that diagnosis.

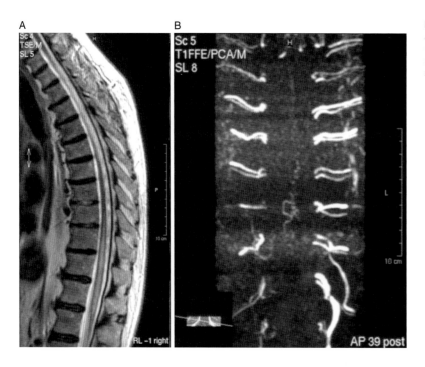

Figure 8.1. (A) T2-weighted MRI showing a large longitudinal hyperintense myelopathy lesion and widened perimedullar veins. (B) MR angiography showing a feeding artery at level T11.

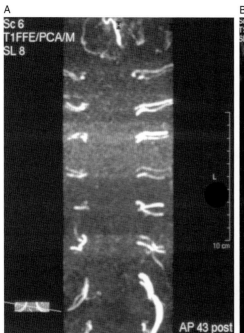
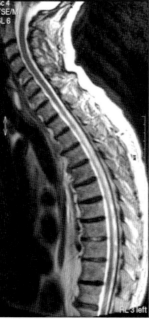

Figure 8.2. (A) Successful embolization of the feeding artery. (B) Thickening of the spinal cord and myelopathy lesion have disappeared four months after embolization.

Follow-up

An MR angiography revealed an SDAVF with a feeding artery at level T11 (Figure 8.1). Embolization was successful (Figure 8.2). Using a walking stick, his walking distance increased; he could continue for 30 minutes. Muscle cramps did not improve. There was no relapse during the follow-up period.

General remarks

The first clinical and pathological description of this syndrome was by Foix and Alajouanine. Since the introduction of spinal MRI, the ability to diagnose SDAVF at earlier stages has dramatically improved. SDAVF manifests predominantly in males with a mean age at diagnosis of between 55 and 60 years.

SDAVFs originate from an abnormal connection between an artery and vein at the level of a dural root sleeve in the intervertebral foramen, with low flow. As they are located outside the spinal parenchyma, SDAVFs do not cause spinal hemorrhages, in contrast to arteriovenous malformations. Over 90% of fistulas are located in the thoracic region.

Diagnostic delay may be 1–4 years. Early symptoms are often nonspecific and include, in a majority of patients:

- gait disturbances
- symmetric or asymmetric sensory disturbances of the legs, such as paresthesias in one or both feet, diffuse or patchy sensory loss
- radicular pain
- complaints of micturition

Some patients have fecal incontinence, sensory loss in the buttocks, or erectile dysfunction. Acute onset with symptoms developing within minutes to hours occurs in a minority of cases. These patients mimic cases with an anterior spinal artery syndrome and not neuromuscular syndromes.

Most patients with SDAVF have chronic disease that may mimic various neuromuscular disorders (Table 8.1). At diagnosis, about 80% of patients have some degree of leg weakness. These include paraparesis and UMN signs in the legs. If untreated, patients develop ascending myelopathy with congestive edema, and ultimately infarction of the caudal end of the spinal cord. Treatment consists of endovascular embolization or surgical ligation of the fistula. Recurrences may occur with either treatment method.

Table 8.1. Differential diagnosis of spinal dural arteriovenous fistula

Disease/ syndrome	Clinical characteristics	EMG and other diagnostic tests
ALS/MND	Distal onset weakness with atrophy UMN signs No sensory signs No sphincter signs Rapid progression (weeks–months)	Denervation more generalized Spine MRI normal
Slowly progressive PMA	Pure motor weakness with atrophy and fasciculation Frequently asymmetric at onset Frequent arm-onset Slow progression (months–years) No sensory signs No sphincter signs	Localized denervation Spine MRI normal
Motor variant of CIDP	Usually symmetric from onset No sphincter signs	Generalized, focal conduction abnormalities: conduction block, slow conduction, prolonged distal motor latencies, abnormal F-waves and H-reflexes
Sensory polyneuropathy	Stocking-and-glove sensory loss Proximal sensory loss at legs and buttocks exceptional Micturition problems not prominent	Abnormal EMG Spine MRI normal
Spinal tumor	Myelopathy, cauda equina syndrome	Spine MRI abnormal
Tethered spinal cord	Can present with radicular pain	Spine MRI abnormal

Suggested reading

Jellema K, Canta LR, Tijssen CC, et al. Spinal dural arterovenous fistulas: clinical features in 80 patients. *J Neurol Neurosurg Psychiatry* 2003; **74**: 1438–1440.

Jellema K, Tijssen CC, Van Gijn J. Spinal dural arteriovenous fistulas: a congestive myelopathy that initially mimics a peripheral nerve disorder. *Brain* 2006; **129**: 3150–3164.

Charcot–Marie–Tooth disease type 1A: a secretary with tingling of the hands

Clinical history

A 46-year-old female complained about having painless tingling of the fingers for about the past 15 years, which was hindering her secretarial work. Initially she noticed these sensations at night; shaking the hands reduced the tingling. Eventually, the symptoms also became apparent while reading or riding a bike. She never noticed tingling of the feet or toes. For about a year she had felt tiredness in her forearms and legs following exertion. She had had "hollow" feet since early childhood, as does her daughter.

She admitted that she had never been keen on sport and had always been a little bit slow compared to her peers.

Examination

Inspection revealed she had pes cavus and a tendency to clawing of the feet. She could not easily walk on her heels due to slight weakness of both anterior tibial muscles. The Achilles tendon reflexes were reduced. Otherwise, the neurological examination was normal.

Ancillary investigations

Nerve conduction studies showed markedly reduced conduction velocities of the motor and sensory nerves consistent with a demyelinating neuropathy. Motor conduction velocity of the ulnar nerve was 27 m/s (normal >50 m/s). DNA analysis revealed a duplication on chromosome 17p. A diagnosis of Charcot–Marie–Tooth (CMT) disease or hereditary motor and sensory neuropathy type 1A could, therefore, be established.

General remarks

CMT disease, first described in 1886, was named after the three clinicians who reported it and is the most common inherited neuromuscular disorder, affecting at least 1 in 2500 persons. In the past, the classification of CMT, also known as hereditary motor and sensory neuropathy (HSMN), was determined by the nature of the peripheral nerve disease; for instance, demyelinating versus axonal type. In order to differentiate between these two basic abnormalities,

electrophysiological or histopathological investigations have been applied. CMT1 disease (demyelinating) and CMT2 disease (axonal) could be distinguished, using upper limb motor nerve conduction velocities (MNCVs) (measured at the median or ulnar nerves), type 1 being defined by having MNCVs <38 m/s and type 2 by MNCVs >38 m/s. There is also an intermediate type, with median or ulnar nerve MNCVs between the demyelinating and axonal range (between 25 and 45 m/s).

Since the identification of the 1.4Mb duplication of chromosome 17 containing the peripheral myelin protein 22 (PMP22) gene as the cause of CMT1A – making PMP22 the first causative gene for CMT to be identified – there have been rapid advances in understanding the molecular basis for many forms of CMT and more than 30 causative genes have been identified to date. A classification purely on the basis of genetic denomination, however, is not desirable as there is considerable genetic heterogeneity. For example, myelin protein zero (MPZ) mutations were originally described as causing autosomal dominant (AD) CMT1 (CMT1B), but are now recognized as causing autosomal recessive (AR) CMT1, AD CMT2, and intermediate CMT as well. In addition to an AD and an AR subtype, one can distinguish an X-linked dominantly inherited form (Case 12).

Clinical features can help the clinician to decide whether a neuropathy is likely to be genetic (Table 9.1). It is important not to rule out an inherited neuropathy if the clinical features raise the possibility, even in the absence of a family history. These apparently sporadic patients are frequently encountered in practice and usually have mutations in the common AD genes including, in some cases, de novo dominant mutations. Mutations in AR genes are less common. A carefully taken family history may help the clinician to refine the diagnosis further. If there is male-to-male transmission, this suggests AD inheritance. If there is no male-to-male transmission, inheritance may still be AD but it can also be an X-linked dominant trait. When taking the history, it is important to include ethnic background, because in countries with a high rate of consanguineous marriages, AR inheritance is more likely.

Table 9.1. Clinical features of a hereditary neuropathy

- Positive family history (can be absent due to the clinical variability)
- Usually early presentation (infancy–adolescence), but in CMT2 onset may be as late as in the seventh decade
- Some CMT1 patients, when adult, only mention complaints from skeletal abnormalities; e.g., scoliosis or pes cavus
- Slow disease progression
- Presence of foot deformities and scoliosis
- In adults: lack of positive sensory symptoms despite clear sensory signs on examination

In most populations, AD CMT1 is the most common form of CMT. Patients usually present with a classic CMT phenotype characterized by walking difficulty and foot deformity (e.g., pes cavus; Figure 9.1), with onset in the first two decades accompanied by distal atrophy, weakness and sensory loss, and hyporeflexia. There is a marked clinical variability, about 10% of cases being asymptomatic or paucisymptomatic like our patient. At the other end of the spectrum (also ~10%), patients are wheelchair-bound. Additionally, atrophy of hand muscles can vary (Figure 9.2). If severe, clawing of the fingers can occur (Figure 9.3). Respiratory insufficiency due to involvement of the diaphragm is very rare.

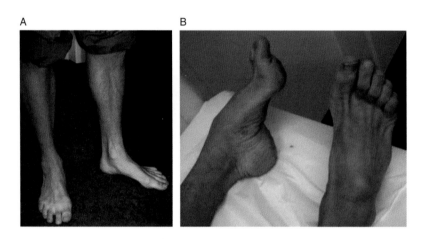

A   B

Figure 9.1. (A, B) Pes cavus in a patient with CMT1A.

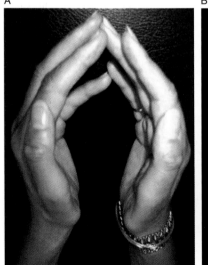
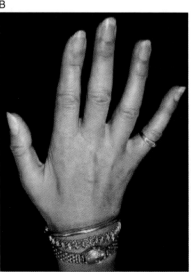

A   B

Figure 9.2. Thenar atrophy (A) and first interosseal dorsal muscle atrophy (B) in a patient with CMT1A.

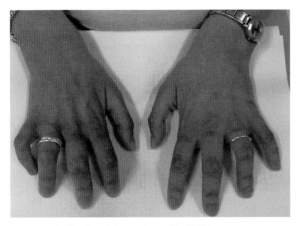

Figure 9.3. Claw hands in a patient with CMT1A.

It is often easier to ascertain the decade of onset rather than the year of onset as the symptoms in the first two decades of life may be nonspecific (e.g., poor at sports, last in races, clumsiness, difficulty with fitting shoes).

The classic CMT phenotype is length dependent, the upper limbs becoming affected later than the lower limbs. Usually, in CMT1A there is diffuse slowing of MNCV. Unless specifically asked about it, it is very common for the patients not to complain of hand weakness, which is detectable on examination. Median and ulnar MNCVs are, by definition, below 38 m/s, the sensory nerve action potentials (SNAPs) being either reduced or absent. As genetic tests are easily available and frequently diagnostic, nerve biopsies are now rarely performed for establishing a diagnosis. Abnormalities that are characteristic in a biopsy, albeit not specific, include demyelination and remyelination, and onion bulb formation.

The approach to the genetic diagnosis of AD CMT1 requires an appreciation of the frequency with which a particular gene may cause AD CMT1. Classic CMT phenotypes and MNCVs less than 38 m/s (commonly around 20 m/s) are strongly suggestive of CMT1A. The lack of family history does not exclude CMT1A, as about 10% of the CMT1A cases are sporadic. In European populations, CMT1A accounts for ~50% of all CMT1 cases. Point mutations in the PMP22 gene can also cause CMT1, but are associated with a wider spectrum of phenotypes, including classic CMT1A and more severe CMT1.

CMT1B is the second most common cause of AD CMT1 and is due to mutations in the MPZ gene comprising about 10% of AD CMT1. Patients can present with the classic CMT1 phenotype but are more likely to have either a more severe early onset form of CMT, with MCV <10 m/s, or a late-onset form of CMT, with median MNCVs in the intermediate (axonal) range.

Mutations in other genes, including lipopolysaccharide-induced tumor necrosis factor (LITAF) and early growth response 2 (EGR2) are rare. Mutations in the former usually cause a classic phenotype, whereas those in the latter give rise to a more severe and young-onset form of CMT. Mutations in the neurofilament light chain polypeptide 68 kDa (NEFL) gene were originally described as a (rare) cause of CMT2, but also need to be considered in patients with AD CMT1.

In general, patients with AR demyelinating CMT, which is classified as CMT4A, B, C, etc., have an early onset of the disease and are more severely affected than patients with classic AD CMT1. Weakness often progresses to involve proximal muscles and may result in early loss of ambulation. Unlike most cases of AD CMT1, nerve biopsies can be a useful addition in phenotyping certain cases, because specific features make a particular genetic diagnosis more likely, albeit that, here too, there can be heterogeneity. Focally folded myelin can be found in myotubularin-related protein 2 (MTMR2), MTMR13, and MPZ-related AR CMT1.

Severe and early scoliosis may be seen with CMT4C due to mutations in the SH3 domain and the tetratricopeptide repeats 2 (SH3TC2) gene. Characteristic nerve biopsy features include basal membrane onion bulbs and multiple cytoplasmic processes of the Schwann cells ensheathing unmyelinated axons.

With regard to the disease course in adult CMT1A patients, cross-sectional studies show that clinical disease severity at the impairment and disability level is related to axonal dysfunction. This was considered to be the cause of the decline in motor function that was previously observed. A five-year follow-up study showed, however, that the decline in adulthood may, to a considerable extent, reflect a process of normal aging rather than ongoing active disease. In the same study, physical disability increased over time in adult patients while controls did not perceive any physical disability.

According to a recent Cochrane review, none of the small trials of exercise, creatine, purified brain gangliosides, or orthoses that have been performed produced significant benefit. Ascorbic acid has not been shown to be beneficial either. In general, the patients are referred to the rehabilitation physician for aids, such as orthopedic shoes, orthoses, cane, or crutches. Surgical interventions are carried out if the foot deformities increase and cannot be corrected by orthopedic shoes.

Suggested reading

Gabreëls-Festen A, van Beersum S, Eshuis L, et al. Study on the gene and phenotypic characterisation of autosomal recessive demyelinating motor and sensory neuropathy (Charcot–Marie–Tooth disease) with a gene locus on chromosome 5q23-q33. *J Neurol Neurosurg Psychiatry* 1999; **66**: 569–574.

Reilly MM, Murphy SM, Laurá M. Charcot–Marie–Tooth disease. *J Peripher Nerv Syst* 2011; **16**: 1–14.

Verhamme C, van Schaik IN, Koelman JH, de Haan RJ, de Visser M. The natural history of Charcot–Marie–Tooth type 1A in adults: a 5-year follow-up study. *Brain* 2009; **132**: 3252–3262.

Young P, De Jonghe P, Stögbauer F, Butterfass-Bahloul T. Treatment for Charcot–Marie–Tooth disease. Cochrane Database Syst Rev 2008; CD006052.

www.molgen.ua.ac.be/CMTMutations; www.musclegene table.fr; www.neuromuscular.wustl.edu

CASE 10

Hereditary neuropathy with liability to pressure palsy: a general practitioner complaining about numbness of the hands

Clinical history

Since the age of 18, this GP, now aged 55 years, had experienced numbness of the hands during cycling and when handling scissors. For about a year, she had noticed weakness of the hand muscles, which restricted her in certain activities such as pumping the cuff for measuring the blood pressure of her patients. She also became aware of wasting of her hand muscles. In addition, she now had permanent tingling of her hands and feet.

The family history is relevant inasmuch as several paternal family members had been diagnosed with hereditary neuropathy with liability to pressure palsy (HNPP). Her daughter has "hollow" feet.

Examination

She was found to have pes cavus and claw toes. There was slight (MRC grade 4–5) weakness of the triceps brachii muscle on the right. Despite bilateral atrophy of the dorsal interosseal muscles and the abductor pollicis, there was no obvious weakness of the hand muscles. She could not walk on her heels due to slight (MRC grade 4–5) weakness of the foot extensor muscles. She had hypesthesia; joint position and vibration sense of the feet were diminished. Muscle tendon reflexes were normal.

Ancillary investigations and diagnostic considerations

EMG and nerve conduction studies had been performed by the referring neurologist. The only significant findings were increased distal motor latencies (DMLs) of the median nerve. DNA analysis revealed a deletion containing the PMP22 gene, on chromosome 17p, which confirmed that she too was diagnosed with HNPP.

Follow-up

She was advised to avoid pressure on nerves close to the surface of the body and not to overstretch nerves.

General remarks

HNPP is an AD inherited disorder; 85% of cases have a deletion identical to the region where, in CMT IA, duplication can be found. In the remaining cases with HNPP, point mutations in the PMP22 gene are causative. More than one-third of the cases have no positive family history. There is reduced penetrance signifying that clinical severity is markedly variable within families. This notion may partly explain the "negative" family history in many cases. However, 20% of patients affected with HNPP and a PMP-22 deletion have a de novo mutation. HNPP is found in ~9% of all genetically defined cases of CMT phenotype.

Age at onset is usually in the second and third decade. Onset in childhood is rare.

Pressure palsies are the hallmark of the disease. Mild trauma or compression is the cause in 40% of patients; other causes are repeated local exercise or stretching. In 10% of cases, symptoms and signs are noticed on waking.

The ulnar and peroneal nerves are most frequently involved but virtually every nerve can be affected. Pressure on the radial nerve may cause transient dropping of the hand or fingers. Even the brachial plexus can be affected. The absence of pain discriminates the condition from idiopathic and hereditary neuralgic amyotrophy, albeit that about 5% of these patients report no pain before the attack. Despite the term palsy, there are usually sensory disturbances, as in our patient, without muscle weakness. Usually the symptoms and signs are mild and transient with full recovery over a period of a few days to months. In due course and with repeated minor nerve injuries, there may be persistent, often asymmetric weakness, especially in the hand. This may cause claw fingers and foot drop. In some advanced cases, the phenotype is close to the classic form of CMT.

If the diagnosis is suspected in a singleton case, based on the history and clinical examination, nerve conduction studies are indicated. Typical cases show prolonged DMLs (except for the tibial nerve), slowing or conduction block of motor nerves at entrapment sites, reduced distal sensory conduction velocity, and reduced SNAP amplitudes. Entrapment sites can be found at the elbow (ulnar nerve) and at the fibular head (peroneal nerve). DNA confirmation is the ultimate proof. In the pregenetic era, nerve biopsies were performed and showed tomacula, a sign of focal thickening of the myelin sheath (Figure 10.1). As in most hereditary neuropathies, sural nerve biopsies are for diagnostic purposes no longer performed when a diagnosis of HNPP is considered.

Therapeutic interventions consist of recommendations to avoid pressure or stretch injury of nerves.

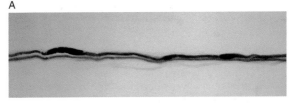

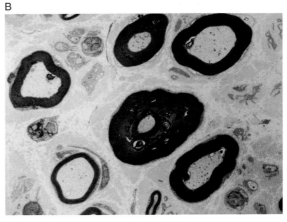

Figure 10.1. Mutation analysis has replaced histopathological diagnosis in most neuropathies where a hereditary cause is considered, such as in HNPP. In the pregenetic era, nerve biopsies were performed for diagnostic purposes. (A) Teased (single) nerve fiber showing tomacula (Latin for sausage)–sausage-shaped focal myelin overgrowth. Hence the old name for HNPP is tomaculous neuropathy. (B) Electron micrograph showing redundant myelin loop formation around the central axon. Lower left: axon with a thin myelin sheath following remyelination (x7000).

These include the advice not to lean with the elbow on hard surfaces (ulnar nerve), not to reach backward with the arm over the hard back of a chair (radial nerve), and not to squat or kneel for any length of time (peroneal nerve). In advanced cases with a CMT-like phenotype, orthopedic shoes or orthoses can be helpful.

Suggested reading

Saporta AS, Sottile SL, Miller LJ, et al. Charcot–Marie–Tooth disease subtypes and genetic testing strategies. *Ann Neurol* 2011; **69**: 22–33.

Charcot–Marie–Tooth disease type 2A, mitofusinopathy: a family with severe neuropathy and atrophy of the optic nerve

Clinical history

The index patient was referred at the age of 40 years because he wished to be informed about the genetic nature of his disorder. He was diagnosed with CMT disease. At 14 months of age, he started walking, but awkwardly due to a bilateral foot drop for which braces were prescribed. On first examination at the age of 2 years and 8 months, there was marked atrophy, hypotonia, and areflexia of the lower legs and slight wasting of the thenar and hypothenar muscles. At that time, nerve conduction studies showed normal MNCVs of arm nerves. No MUPs could be recorded in the lower leg muscles on concentric needle EMG.

Weakness and atrophy were progressive, leading to wheelchair dependency at the age of 11 years. For a long time, it was known that he had decreased vision and had complaints about the quality of his voice. He had no other symptoms, in particular, no breathlessness.

The family history disclosed that his father, who died at age 63 years, probably due to respiratory insufficiency, had been evaluated in our hospital at the age of 35 years with an identical clinical picture. He started to walk at 14 months of age, but his gait had always been clumsy. Progression was relentless and he became wheelchair-bound by the age of 14 years. Examination was similar to that described in his son, consisting of bilateral opticopathy with marked decreased visual acuity of 2/60 and severe wasting, weakness, and contractures of all four limbs. The father had left-sided strabismus divergens with limited adduction. In addition, he had severe sensory disturbances and generalized areflexia.

Similarly, the older brother of the index patient was affected with an identical clinical picture of polyneuropathy and opticopathy. In addition, he was found to have bilateral vocal cord paralysis. From the age of 42 years he had received nocturnal non-invasive ventilatory support. At 43 years old, he died unexpectedly, probably due to pneumonia.

Examination

On examination at age 40 years, the patient had a high-pitched and hoarse voice, decreased movement of the vocal cords, marked atrophy and weakness of the arms and legs, distal more than proximal, with contractures of the major joints and the finger flexors, scapulae alatae ("winged" scapulae), pectus excavatum ("hollowed" chest), marked lumbar hyperlordosis, and a scoliosis.

He had marked distal sensory disturbances, with absent position sense of toes and fingers, and generalized areflexia.

Ophthalmological examination revealed a visual acuity of 4/20. There was mild anisocoria, the left pupil being slightly larger, that did not change according to the degree of light. The pupillary reactions were slow and symmetric. There were no ocular motility disturbances. Ophthalmoscopic examination revealed very pale optic discs with a small cup. The macula, peripheral retina, and blood vessels were normal.

Ancillary investigations

Additional investigation with electrophysiology showed an abnormal visual evoked potential (VEP). The pattern of the VEP was flat, and with a flash VEP, very weak responses were elicited. The electroretinogram was normal. It was concluded that there was a severe optic atrophy that had been stable for at least 13 years.

VC was decreased (62% of expected). EMG showed severe axonal sensorimotor polyneuropathy with absent CMAPs and SNAPs of the distal nerves of arms and legs.

DNA analysis revealed a missense mutation (c.1090C>T, p.R364W) in the mitofusin 2 (MFN2) gene on chromosome 1p36.2.

Diagnostic considerations

Owing to the genetic findings, a diagnosis of axonal neuropathy with optic atrophy caused by mutations in mitofusin 2 could be established.

Table 11.1. Phenotypes of Charcot–Marie–Tooth disease type 2 (AD, X-linked dominant, sporadic)

- Motor and sensory neuropathy: CMT2A (MFN2), X-CMT (GJB1), CMT2I/J (MPZ)

- Sensory neuropathy with ulceromutilations: CMT2B (RAB7 gene). Carefully evaluate the toes for ulcers. Patients may have had amputations (Figure 11.2)

- Motor neuropathy/distal spinal muscular atrophy (BSCL2, HSP1, HSP8)

BSCL2, see Case 3.

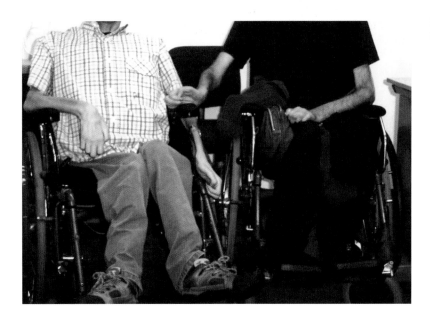

Figure 11.1. Two brothers with CMT2A caused by a MFN2 mutation.

General remarks

Historically, CMT neuropathies have been divided according to neuropathological and electrophysiological criteria into demyelinating CMT1 (Case 9) and axonal CMT2. CMT2 can be subdivided into three distinct phenotypes (Table 11.1). In the first and most common phenotype, patients present with the classic CMT picture – muscle atrophy and weakness and sensory disturbances of the lower legs and hands, often associated with pes cavus – although sometimes the phenotype may be earlier or later than usually seen with CMT1A (Figure 11.1). Patients with this form of the CMT2 phenotype are indistinguishable from CMT1 without neurophysiological examination.

The second phenotype is predominantly sensory CMT disease, called type 2B, caused by RAB7 mutations (Figure 11.2). The third group consists of patients with prominent motor involvement, often leading to confusion about whether the disorder is CMT2 or distal hereditary motor neuropathy. In the latter group, the phenotype is often similar to that of CMT without sensory disturbances.

CMT disease type 2A (CMT2A), caused by mutations in the MFN2 gene, comprises about 20% of patients with the classic CMT phenotype. There is clinical heterogeneity with mild cases at one end of the spectrum, and at the other end, severe cases with children requiring wheelchairs. In some pedigrees, CMT2 is known to be associated with a variety of

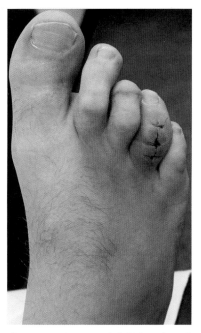

Figure 11.2. Patient with CMT2B in whom the distal part of his third digit of the right foot was amputated because of poorly healing ulcers and osteomyelitis. He recently underwent surgery for another ulcer.

additional symptoms, such as spastic paraparesis or optic atrophy. Axonal CMT with optic atrophy caused by MFN2 mutations, as found in the case report, is referred to as HSMN type VI or CMT VI.

51

Recently, mutations in the dynamin 2 gene have also been implicated with AD CMT disease. This disease had been called CMT disease type B. Patients have a classic CMT phenotype with mild to moderate severity, as less than 5% of patients are wheelchair-bound. Age at onset may range between two and 50 years. MNCV may be in the axonal range with mild reduction, or be intermediate. Early onset cataract has been observed in families with CMTB disease.

Suggested reading

Claeys KG, Züchner S, Kennerson M, et al. Phenotypic spectrum of dynamin-2 mutations in Charcot–Marie–Tooth neuropathy. *Brain* 2009; **132**: 1741–1752.

Shy ME, Patzkó A. Axonal Charcot–Marie–Tooth disease. *Curr Opin Neurol* 2011; **24**: 475–483.

Züchner S, De Jonghe P, Jordanova A, et al. Axonal neuropathy with optic atrophy is caused by mutations in mitofusin 2. *Ann Neurol* 2006; **59**: 276–281.

CASE 12 · X-linked Charcot–Marie–Tooth disease: a middle-aged designer with progressive walking difficulty

Clinical history

At the age of 49 years, this man was referred by his GP. It had been known for quite some time that he had wasting of the hand muscles, which urged him to use the computer more often for his design activities. An increase in the frequency of stumbling made him seek medical help.

His medical history revealed that he was a late walker and that, as a child, he had always had difficulty running. His mother, who was deceased, was apparently asymptomatic, but two maternal nephews, known to our hospital, were diagnosed with an as yet unclassified axonal type of Charcot–Marie–Tooth (CMT2) disease.

Examination

There was atrophy of the interosseal muscles, the thenar muscles, and the lower legs (Figure 12.1). He had pes cavus and claw toes. He walked with a steppage gait and was not able to tiptoe. Muscle strength testing revealed paralysis of the anterior tibial muscles, and severe symmetric weakness of his toe extensors and calf muscles. There were sensory abnormalities in the lower legs. He had a fine postural hand tremor. Arm reflexes were hypoactive and leg reflexes were absent.

His maternal nephews were less severely affected; their calf muscles were hypertrophic.

Ancillary investigations

We did not perform nerve conduction studies in our patient as one of his maternal nephews had already been examined. MNCV of the ulnar nerve was mildly decreased with slowing not fulfilling criteria for demyelination (43 m/s). This excludes CMT type 1A due to a PMP 22 duplication (Case 9). DNA analysis of the gap junction beta 1 (GJB1) or connexin 32 gene on chromosome Xq13.1 was carried out and a c.-103C>T mutation at the 5'UTR end of the gene was identified.

Diagnostic considerations

A diagnosis of X-linked dominant CMT could be made on the basis of the genetic finding.

General remarks

CMTX1, an X-linked dominant disorder, caused by mutations in the GJB1 gene is the second most common form of CMT. As expected in an X-linked disorder, males are usually more severely affected than females. Males usually present with symptoms in the first two decades of life, with lower leg wasting and weakness. Foot deformities are observed in almost all patients. Most patients have distal sensory loss of all modalities and areflexia of the lower limbs. Although the neuropathy is essentially length dependent, frequently some asymmetry, such as various degrees of ankle dorsiflexion weakness, is evident. This may discriminate CMTX1 from the classic CMT phenotype of CMT1A.

The phenotype in females shows more variation and includes asymptomatic patients in whom signs are only found on examination. This is postulated to be due to random X-inactivation. Females carry two copies of the X chromosome, resulting in a potentially toxic double dose of X-linked genes. To correct this

A   B   C

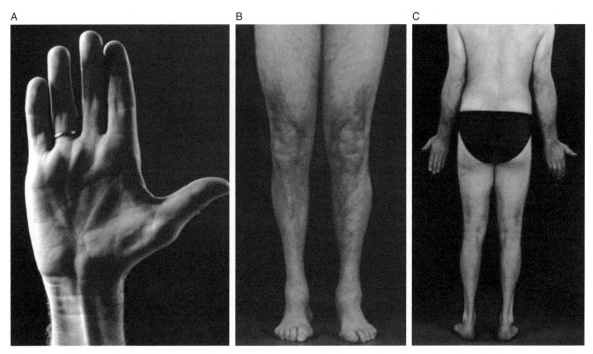

Figure 12.1. Patient with CMTX. (A) Atrophy of the thenar and intrinsic muscles. Owing to intrinsic muscle weakness, the fingers cannot be kept together. (B, C) Atrophy of lower leg muscles, more pronounced in the right leg.

imbalance, mammalian females have evolved a unique mechanism of dosage compensation. By way of the process called X-chromosome inactivation, female mammals transcriptionally silence one of their two X chromosomes in a complex and highly coordinated manner. The choice of which X chromosome will be inactivated is random.

In both males and females, the MNCVs are usually in the intermediate range (25–40 m/s) compared with much lower values in demyelinating CMT1. Nerve conduction is commonly slower in males compared to females with values in the upper range of demyelinating CMT1. Nerve conduction in females is usually in the axonal CMT2 range. There is a variable spectrum with mild cases, like our patient (43 m/s falling in the axonal range), and wheelchair-bound cases with onset <10 years of age and very low MNCVs.

Patients may have mild asymptomatic involvement of the central nervous system (CNS) (e.g., extensor plantar responses, mild deafness, abnormal brainstem-evoked potentials). Occasionally, transient severe CNS involvement characterized by ataxia and dysarthria has been described, associated with nonenhancing, confluent, symmetric lesions in the white matter and corpus callosum.

Suggested reading

Dubourg O, Tardieu S, Birouk N, et al. Clinical, electrophysiological and molecular genetic chracteristics of 93 patients with X-linked Charcot–Marie–Tooth disease. *Brain* 2004; **124**: 1958–1967.

Reilly MM, Murphy SM, Laurá M. Charcot–Marie–Tooth disease. *J Peripher Nerv Syst* 2011; **16**: 1–14.

Hereditary sensory and autonomic neuropathy type 4: two sisters with spontaneous bone fractures that caused little pain

Clinical history

Within a period of a few days, a 34-year-old woman of Moroccan descent developed progressive weakness of the right leg without pain. Having suffered spontaneous bone fractures as a child, she had been diagnosed with insensitivity to pain syndrome. She had never been able to perspire; this meant warm weather was not well tolerated and it resulted in an increase in body temperature.

Her 36-year-old sister also suffered several spontaneous bone fractures without pain. She had similar but less severe complaints. The parents are full cousins.

Examination

The patient was of short stature. Sharp–dull discrimination was diminished in the arms, more pronounced distally. Passive movements of the legs caused some back pain. Muscle strength and pain sense in the right leg were diminished. Below the knees, sharp–dull discrimination was absent and warm–cold sensation disturbed. Vibration sense was normal. She had Charcot deformities, neuropathic arthropathy of the right knee and ankle (Figure 13.1, Table 13.1). Owing to sensory disturbances, microtrauma and the resulting inflammatory response passed unnoticed. Autonomic dysregulation may play an additional role. Bone resorption causes deformity of a joint. The tip of the right thumb had been amputated following panaritium.

Ancillary examination

The MRI scan of the lumbosacral spine showed collapse of the first and second lumbar vertebrae compatible with neurogenic arthropathy. In addition, the MRI of the cervical spine showed neurogenic arthropathy at the level C4–C7 (Figure 13.2).

Follow-up

After decompression and fixation of the spine, muscle strength improved. Four years later, she complained of stiffness when walking, altered feeling and decreased strength in both hands, and tingling in the fingertips that progressed over periods of weeks. A cervical MRI showed severe degeneration of cervical vertebrae leading to spinal stenosis and myelopathy. She had no pyramidal signs. Following C3–C6 cervical laminectomy and spondylodesis, her neurological condition improved.

Needle EMG and motor nerve conduction studies were normal. SNAPs were reduced in arm nerves and could not be elicited in lower limb nerves, suggesting dying back axonal degeneration. Short stimuli of 30 mA caused pain.

Neurological examination of the sister showed completely normal pain sensation in the arms with decreased pain sense below the knees.

Table 13.1. Charcot deformity of joints, syndrome. Charcot arthropathy, Charcot neuropathic arthropathy, neuro-osteoarthropathy (JM Charcot, 1868)

Causes

Myelopathies
- Syringomyelia
- Spina bifida
- Trauma
- Tabes dorsalis

Neuropathies
- Diabetes mellitus
- Leprosy
- HSAN
- CMT disease (extremely rare)

Symptoms
- Erythema, edema, elevated temperature of the affected joint
- Pain (can be absent in HSAN)
- Thickening of the joint
- Deformity of the joint
- Loss of function
- Crepitation at palpation

Pathogenesis: repeat (minor) trauma causes joint damage that goes unnoticed in patients with loss of pain sense with or without loss of proprioception. Infective osteomyelitis, as may be a consequence of concomitant skin ulcers, is not obligatory. Joint effusion, hydrarthrosis, synovial hypertrophy, and capsular thickening with granulomatous tissue and florid ossification may follow. Subluxations and periarticular fractures will cause deformity of joints. Initially, a plain radiograph can be normal. Early recognition and immobilization can help to prevent deformity.

Diagnostic considerations

DNA analysis revealed two homozygous mutations in the NTRK 1 gene, confirming a diagnosis of hereditary sensory and autonomic neuropathy (HSAN) type 4. These mutations target the domain for the neurotrophin tyrosine kinase receptor.

General remarks

Both sisters had neuropathy with congenital insensitivity to pain, decreased cold and warm sensation and anhidrosis, and skin ulcers ("panaritium"). Proprioception, muscle strength, and reflexes were normal. Early onset with fractures and consanguinity of the parents suggested AR HSAN. Heredity of eight known HSAN can be AD or AR. Currently, seven genes have been implicated. Some patients also have clinical or electrophysiological motor abnormalities, showing overlap between HSAN and CMT disease. RAB7 mutations cause AD CMT2B neuropathy with skin ulcers (Table 11.1). HSAN with predominant or pure dysautonomia is called the Railey–Day syndrome. Skin ulcers and chronic osteomyelitis may necessitate amputations. The tyrosine kinase receptor supports survival of sympathetic ganglion

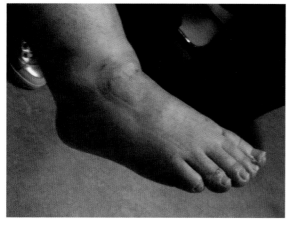

Figure 13.1. Charcot deformity of the right foot in a patient with HSAN.

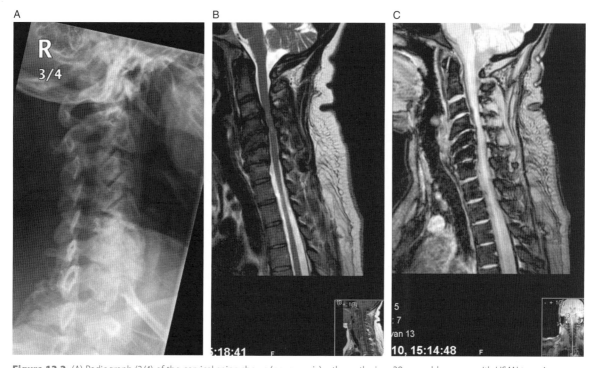

Figure 13.2. (A) Radiograph (3/4) of the cervical spine shows (neurogenic) arthropathy in a 38-year-old woman with HSAN type 4. At the C5–C7 level, sclerosis and abnormal bone deposition at the intervertebral joints can be observed. (B) T2-weighted MRI scan shows loss of height of the 4th, 5th, and 6th cervical vertebrae with abnormal bone formation causing cervical stenosis and a myelopathy lesion. (C) T2-weighted fast-field echo showing abnormal bone formation around the 4th to 6th cervical vertebrae.

neurons and nociceptive (pain and temperature) sensors in the dorsal root ganglions.

Suggested reading

Bruckner FE, Howell A. Neuropathic joints. *Semin Arthritis Rheum* 1972; **2**: 47–69.

Rotthier A, Baets J, De Vriendt E, et al. Genes for hereditary sensory and autonomic neuropathies: a genotype–phenotype correlation. *Brain* 2009; **132**: 2699–2711.

www.molgen.ua.ac.be/CMTMutations

CASE 14 Guillain–Barré syndrome: a sportsman who could no longer run

Clinical history

A 20-year-old, previously healthy student noticed that he was unable to run. The next day he could not walk up stairs and lost strength in his arms. He was admitted to hospital and within the next few hours he progressively lost muscle power in his arms and legs. He did not complain about double vision, but swallowing became progressively impaired. He did have minor tingling and a dull feeling in both hands and feet, but no other sensory complaints. One week prior to admission, he had had a minor upper respiratory tract infection.

Examination

The patient was slightly short of breath and could barely walk. Initially, he was admitted to the neurology ward. Cranial nerve examination revealed a mild bilateral facial palsy, but no other abnormalities. There was a severe paresis of the muscles of arms and legs, proximal MRC grade 4, distal grade 3. He had minor sensory abnormalities in both hands and in the legs, distally from his knees. These consisted of decreased pinprick and tactile sensation and shortened vibration sense. He had areflexia and normal plantar reflexes. Over the next few hours, weakness worsened and respiration became more difficult. VC declined to 1.2 L (normal value >4 L). Within four hours of admission, the patient was transferred to the intensive care unit (ICU) for invasive ventilation.

Ancillary investigations

The standard laboratory investigation was normal. CSF examination showed a slightly increased total protein level (0.6 g/L, <0.45) without a cell increase. Electrophysiology, performed two weeks after onset of weakness, showed extremely low compound muscle action potentials and nonrecordable sensory action potentials, compatible with a severe axonal degeneration of motor and sensory nerves. Motor and sensory nerve conduction velocities were within the normal range.

Diagnostic considerations

The diagnosis of GBS was made. Clinically, he had the predominant motor variety, with clear sensory disturbances.

Follow-up

Because of very rapid progression and severe weakness, treatment with IVIg (0.4 g/kg body weight for five consecutive days) was started immediately. We discussed the condition with the patient and told him it was likely that he would need ventilatory support for some time, but that paralysis should be transient and muscle power would return. In the meantime, swallowing became more difficult and weakness progressed. Although he had required artificial ventilation within 24 hours of admission, he could be weaned from the ventilator after eight days and made a very good recovery. After a few weeks, he was discharged to a rehabilitation center, and within two months after onset he could walk upstairs. He made a complete recovery within three months. Fortunately he did not have pain during the course of the disease. He did not suffer from fatigue.

General remarks

The diagnosis of GBS is usually fairly straightforward (Table 14.1). One to two weeks prior to the onset of weakness, most of the patients have an antecedent infection (such as diarrhea or an upper respiratory

Table 14.1. Criteria for the diagnosis of typical Guillain–Barré syndrome

Features required for diagnosis:
- Progressive weakness in both arms and both legs
- Areflexia

Features strongly supporting diagnosis:
- Progression of symptoms over a period of days to four weeks
- Relative symmetry of symptoms
- Mild sensory symptoms or signs
- Cranial nerve involvement, especially bilateral weakness of facial muscles
- Recovery beginning 2–4 wk after progression ceases
- Autonomic dysfunction
- Absence of fever at onset
- High concentration of protein in cerebrospinal fluid, with $<10 \times 10^6$ cells/L
- Typical electrodiagnostic features
- Pain

Features excluding diagnosis:
- Diagnosis of botulism, myasthenia gravis, poliomyelitis, or toxic neuropathy
- Abnormal porphyrin metabolism
- Recent diphtheria
- Purely sensory syndrome, without weakness

Adapted from Asbury AK, Cornblath DR. Assessment of current diagnostic criteria for Guillain–Barré syndrome. *Ann Neurol* 1990; **27**: S21–S24.

tract infection). A role for *Campylobacter jejuni* infection has been firmly established in patients with preceding gastrointestinal tract infections (see Case 15). Acute pain resulting from inflammation of nerves and nerve roots may precede paresis in GBS and thus delay the diagnosis. Patients may complain of sensory disturbances and cranial muscle weakness, and frequently have facial palsy, ophthalmoplegia, or swallowing difficulties. By definition, weakness is progressive over a maximum period of four weeks, but most patients have reached their nadir within two weeks. About 25% of GBS patients admitted to hospital require artificial ventilation for some time. If ophthalmoplegia and sensory ataxia are prominent initial signs, Miller–Fisher syndrome, a variant of GBS, can be diagnosed (Case 15).

After the progressive phase, there is a stationary phase generally ranging from weeks to months, followed by a recovery phase (Figure 14.1). Other causes of rapidly progressive weakness (such as hypophosphatemia, vitamin B1 deficiency, porphyria, rhabdomyolysis, polymyositis, myasthenia gravis, botulism, or poliomyelitis) have to be ruled out, or found to be improbable. CSF examination is helpful as an increased protein level (>1 g/L) without marked cellular reaction suggests GBS. The CSF protein content, however, is often normal in the first week. A CSF cellular reaction ($>50 \times 10^6$ cells/L) practically excludes GBS and may suggest Lyme disease, other causes of chronic meningitis, or leptomeningeal malignancy.

Electrophysiology may distinguish between acute inflammatory demyelinating polyneuropathy (AIDP),

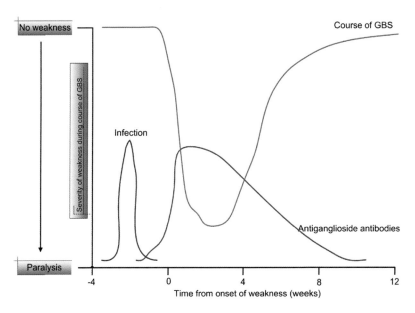

Figure 14.1. Time course of events in patients with GBS. The majority of cases start with a common infection. Progressive weakness develops rapidly followed by a plateau phase of variable duration after which improvement starts. A proportion of patients, especially those with acute motor axonal neuropathy, develop antibodies against the ganglioside GM1. Miller–Fisher syndrome patients very frequently develop antibodies against the ganglioside GQ1b.

the most frequent form of GBS in Europe and the U.S., and the axonal forms of acute motor axonal neuropathy (AMAN) and acute motor and sensory axonal neuropathy (AMSAN), which were found to be more frequent in Japan and China. The prognosis of these predominant axonal neuropathies is not always worse compared with AIDP. In AMAN cases, there is evidence for invasion of macrophages in the periaxonal

space. Many patients have antibodies against the GM1 or GD1a ganglioside (Figure 14.2).

Treatment and prognosis

Good general medical care is essential to prevent aspiration pneumonia, thrombosis, and emergency intubation. Table 14.2 presents a scheme as a possible guide

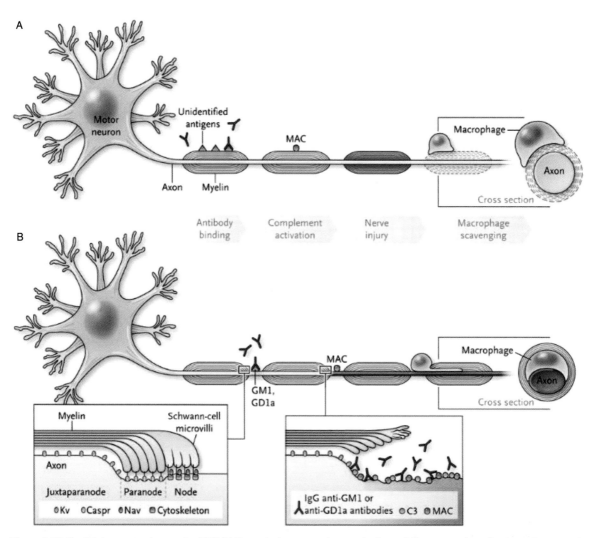

Figure 14.2. Possible immunopathogenesis of GBS. (A) Shows the immunopathogenesis of acute inflammatory demyelinating polyneuropathy (AIDP). Autoantibodies may bind to myelin antigens and activate complement. This is followed by the formation of membrane-attack complex (MAC) on the outer surface of the Schwann cells and the initiation of vesicular degeneration. Macrophages subsequently invade the myelin and act as scavengers to remove myelin debris. (B) Shows the immunopathogenesis of acute motor axonal neuropathy (AMAN). Gangliosides GM1 and GD1a are strongly expressed at the nodes of Ranvier, where the voltage-gated sodium (Nav) channels are localized. Contactin-associated protein (Caspr) and voltage-gated potassium (Kv) channels, respectively, are present at the paranodes and juxtaparanodes. IgG anti-GM1 or anti-GD1a autoantibodies bind to the nodal axolemma, leading to MAC formation. This results in the disappearance of Nav clusters and the detachment of paranodal myelin, which can lead to nerve conduction failure and muscle weakness. Axonal degeneration may follow at a later stage. Macrophages subsequently invade from the nodes into the periaxonal space, scavenging the injured axons (from Yuki N, Hartung H-P. Guillain-Barré syndrome. *New Engl J Med* 2012; **366**: 2294–2304, with permission).

Table 14.2. Monitoring a patient with Guillain–Barré syndrome

Good general medical care

Monitor progression, prevent and manage potentially fatal complications, in particular:
- Regularly monitor pulmonary function (vital capacity, respiration frequency) initially every 2–4 hr; in stable phase, every 6–12 hr
- Regularly check for autonomic dysfunction (blood pressure, heart rate, pupils, peristalsis): continuously monitor pulse and blood pressure (initially alternative every 2–4 hr; in stable phase every 6–12 hr)
- Check for swallowing dysfunction
- Recognize and treat pain: acute neuropathic pain according to WHO guideline, but try to avoid opioids; chronic neuropathic pain, amitriptyline or antiepileptic drugs (e.g., pregabaline, gabapentin)
- Prevent and treat infections and pulmonary embolism
- Prevent cornea ulceration due to facial weakness
- Prevent decubitus and contractures

Consider specific treatment with IVIg or plasma exchange (PE)
- Indication for initiating IVIg or PE: severely affected patients (inability to walk unaided = GBS disability scale ≥3). Start preferably within first two weeks of onset
- IVIg: 0.4g/kg for five days (not known whether 1.0g/kg for two days gives better results); PE: standard 5 x PE with total exchange of five plasma volumes
- Also consider treatment in patients with GBS disability scale 2 who continue to get worse
- Not known whether IVIg is effective in mildly affected patients (GBS disability scale ≤2) or in MFS patients

Indication for re-treatment with IVIg: secondary deterioration after initial improvement or stabilization (treatment-related fluctuation): re-treat with IVIg 0.4g/kg for five days. This advice reflects practical experience as the effect of IVIg for treatment-related fluctuations has not been investigated in an randomized controlled trial (RCT)

Indication for ICU admission
- Rapid progressive severe weakness often with impaired respiration (VC <20 mL/kg)
- Necessity for artificial ventilation
- Insufficient swallowing with high chance of pulmonary infection
- Severe autonomic dysfunction

Prognostic factors related to high chance of respiratory insufficiency
- Rapid progression of weakness (limited number of days between onset and admission)
- Low MRC sumscore (six muscle groups; two-sided; range 0–60)
- Presence of facial and/or bulbar weakness

Fluctuations during course of disease or continued slow progression during 4–8 weeks
- Consider treatment-related fluctuation: repeat treatment
- Consider acute-onset CIDP (A-CIDP) and treat accordingly

Rehabilitation and fatigue
- Start physical therapy early during course of disease
- Start rehabilitation as soon as improvement starts

Adapted from Van Doorn PA, Ruts L, Jacobs BC. Clinical features, pathogenesis, and treatment of Guillain–Barré syndrome. *Lancet Neurol* 2008; **7**: 939–950.

to when and how to monitor GBS patients when admitted to the general neurology ward or the ICU. Two treatments that have proved – apparently equally – effective in patients with GBS are IVIg (0.4 g/kg body weight for five days) or plasma exchange (PE; four sessions of 1–1.5 plasma volume in about two weeks). It has been shown that IVIg is effective in patients who are unable to walk, if started within the first two weeks of onset of weakness, when the disease process is still active. About 10% of GBS patients initially improve, or stabilize after IVIg and then deteriorate again (treatment-related fluctuation). These

patients need a repeat course of IVIg treatment. IVIg is readily available in most countries, does not require special equipment, and seems safer in patients with autonomic failure.

Not all patients, however, improve sufficiently and about 20% are still unable to walk unaided six months after onset. New studies, therefore, are investigating whether patients with a poor prognosis might benefit from a second IVIg dose early in the course of the disease. A very simple clinical prognostic scale can be used to predict the chance of requiring artificial ventilation at hospital admission: the Erasmus GBS

Respiratory Insufficiency Scale (EGRIS). The following parameters are required: duration between onset of weakness and hospital admission, the presence of facial and/or bulbar weakness, and severity of muscle weakness as expressed by a MRC sumscore of six muscle pairs on both sides of the body. Rapidly progressive weakness, facial and/or bulbar weakness, and severe weakness of the limbs all indicate a higher chance of the patient becoming dependent on artificial ventilation. The scale can be a help to decide whether ICU admission is indicated, or the patient can be safely admitted to a general neurology ward.

With the modified Erasmus GBS Outcome Scale (mEGOS), the chance of being able to walk unaided after four weeks, three or six months can be predicted. This scale can be used one week after hospital admission. Indicators for a poor prognosis are: advanced age, presence of diarrhea before onset of weakness, and a higher level of disability using the GBS disability scale. mEGOS may help to develop better treatment strategies for GBS and for counseling and rehabilitation of a GBS patient.

Despite current immunological treatment, the majority of GBS patients do have pain and many remain fatigued for a long period of time. The cause of pain may be neuropathic and result from peripheral nerve sprouting with ephaptic transmission following axonal regeneration, or may be musculoskeletal.

A substantial number of patients develop autonomic disturbances (such as fluctuating blood pressure, heart rhythm disturbances (Table 38.1), or ileus) in the acute phase of the disease. New treatments or treatment schedules for GBS should also focus on these issues (Table 14.2).

Suggested reading

Asbury AK, Cornblath DR. Assessment of current diagnostic criteria for Guillain–Barré syndrome. *Ann Neurol* 1990; **27**: S21–S24.

Patwa HS, Chaudry V, Katzberg H, Rae-Grant AD, So YT. Evidence-based guideline: intravenous immunoglobulin in the treatment of neuromuscular disorders. Report of the Therapeutics and Technology Assessment Subcommittee of the American Academy of Neurology. *Neurology* 2012; **79**: 1009–1015.

Van Doorn PA, Ruts L, Jacobs BC. Clinical features, pathogenesis, and treatment of Guillain–Barré syndrome. *Lancet Neurol* 2008; **7**: 939–950.

Walgaard C, Lingsma HF, Ruts L, et al. Prediction of respiratory insufficieny in Guillain–Barré syndrome. *Ann Neurol* 2010; **67**: 781–787.

Walgaard C, Lingsma HF, Ruts L, et al. Early recognition of poor prognosis in Guillain–Barré syndrome. *Neurology* 2011; **76**: 968–975.

Yuki N, Hartung H-P. Guillain–Barré syndrome. *New Engl J Med* 2012; **366**: 2294–2304.

CASE 15   Miller–Fisher syndrome: walking like a drunk

Clinical history

A 58-year-old, previously healthy man noticed one day that he could no longer walk in a straight line. The next day he was asked whether he was drunk. He noticed that single objects appeared to be double, and at that time, he was almost unable to walk unaided. He said that he drank about 1–2 glasses of alcohol per day. He had had diarrhoea two weeks before onset of these symptoms.

Examination

The patient walked with a wide gait and was very unstable. He had ophthalmoplegia and double vision in all directions (Video 13). He had no other cranial nerve abnormalities and no dysarthria. There was no weakness of the muscles of the arms or legs, no sensory disturbances, but he had areflexia of both arms and legs. The finger–nose test and the knee–heel test were clearly abnormal (ataxia). In addition, he had a severe gait ataxia.

Ancillary investigations

Routine blood and CSF examinations were normal. No distinct abnormalities were revealed by EMG. He tested positively for antibodies to the ganglioside GQ1b.

Diagnostic considerations

Because of the combination of ataxia, ophthalmoplegia, and areflexia, a clinical diagnosis of Miller–Fisher syndrome (MFS) was reached. The absence of antecedent signs of food poisoning and the presence of ataxia exclude botulism. The presence of antibodies to GQ1b after a period of a few weeks further established this diagnosis. In general, it is considered that patients with MFS have a relatively favorable prognosis. As treatment with IVIg has not been shown to be effective in MFS, this was not initiated.

Follow-up

Two days later, however, the patient developed a bilateral facial palsy and some weakness of the extremities. Because of this clear deterioration in the early course of disease, an MFS–GBS overlap syndrome was suggested and IVIg treatment was started (0.4 g/kg body weight for five days). Over a period of six weeks, the patient made an almost complete recovery. When he was discharged he could walk unaided and ophthalmoplegia had disappeared. Areflexia was still present. A few months later he had made a full recovery.

General remarks

MFS is a subgroup (cranial nerve variant) of GBS. Patients with MFS, however, may have symptoms other than ophthalmolegia, ataxia, and areflexia, and there can be an overlap with GBS. Ataxia can be so severe that the patient is bed-ridden (Video 8). In general, it seems that MFS patients with the classic triad of symptoms have a relatively favorable prognosis.

Currently, there are no results available of an RCT that has studied the effect of IVIg treatment in MFS. Therefore, embarking on IVIg treatment is, in general, not recommended in patients with MFS. But it can be considered if the signs are severe, and especially when there is overlap with GBS. Over 80% of patients with MFS have antibodies to the ganglioside GQ1b. These antibodies, however, can also be found in GBS patients with ocular motor disturbances and in patients with Bickerstaff brainstem encephalitis, but not in patients with other (nonimmunological) causes of cranial nerve dysfunction.

Just as in GBS, MFS is often preceded by an infection such as *Campylobacter jejuni* that induces diarrhoea. *C. jejuni* isolates from GBS and MFS patients express lipo-oligosaccharides (LOS) that mimic the carbohydrates of gangliosides present in peripheral nerves. A Campylobacter gene cluster enables some *C. jejuni* isolates to synthesize these specific structures. Specific *C. jejuni* gene variants are essential for the expression of ganglioside-like LOS. The type of ganglioside mimicry in *C. jejuni* seems to determine the specificity of the anti-ganglioside antibodies and the associated variant in GBS. Antibodies in GBS patients (especially anti-GM1) or in MFS (often anti-GQ1b) are usually cross-reactive, and recognize Campylobacter LOS as well as gangliosides or ganglioside complexes. These gangliosides are present abundantly in the peripheral nervous system. Variation in the preceding type of infection, patients' immune response, but also differences in the presence of specific gangliosides between various nerve constituents may explain, at least in part, why some patients develop GBS, and more specifically, why some patients get GBS or MFS. GQ1b is highly expressed in oculomotor nerves, which may explain ophthalmoplegia in MFS. The generation of these cross-reactive antibodies is an example of molecular mimicry between specific microbial antigens and peripheral- or cranial nerve constituents. MFS, like GBS, generally occurs only once in a lifetime. It is important to realize that the triad of areflexia, ataxia, and opthalmoplegia is not always complete. Some patients have a GBS–MFS overlap syndrome. The initial diagnosis can be difficult, especially when there is also involvement of other cranial nerves, or when there is pain. Determining the presence of GQ1b antibodies can facilitate the diagnosis.

Suggested reading

Overell JR, Hsieh ST, Odaka M, Yuki N, Willison HJ. Treatment for Fisher syndrome, Bickerstaff's brainstem encephalitis and related disorders. *Cochrane Database Syst Rev* 2007; **1**: CD004761.

Willison HJ, Yuki N. Peripheral neuropathies and anti-glycolipid antibodies. *Brain* 2002; **125**: 2591–2625.

Yuki N. Fisher syndrome and Bickerstaff brainstem encephalitis (Fisher–Bickerstaff syndrome). *J Neuroimmunol* 2009; **215**: 1–9.

Chronic inflammatory demyelinating polyneuropathy: an active, retired man who could no longer cycle

Clinical history

A previously healthy, very active 68-year-old man, who usually cycled over 100 km several times a week, noticed progressive tingling in his feet and lower legs that increased over a period of several weeks. This was followed by progressive weakness in the arms and legs. After three months, the weakness became so severe that he could not walk without help. He did not use drugs or drink alcohol.

Examination

A general physical examination revealed no abnormalities. He had no cranial nerve abnormalities. He had a symmetric paresis of his arms, MRC grade 4. There was proximal weakness of the legs, grade 3, which was worse compared to the weakness in his lower legs and feet (grade 4). Touch and pain sense were diminished distally from the elbows and knees. Vibration sense had disappeared up to the level of the hips. He had areflexia.

Ancillary investigations

Routine serological examination, including thyroid stimulating hormone (TSH), revealed no abnormalities. In particular, his glucose level was normal and there was no evidence of monoclonal (M) protein. Nerve conduction studies showed a motor and sensory demyelinating polyneuropathy compatible with chronic inflammatory demyelinating polyneuropathy (CIDP). Motor nerve conduction abnormalities included prolonged DMLs consistent with demyelination, conduction velocities consistent with demyelination, and increased temporal dispersion. Slowing of motor nerve conduction was nonuniform. CSF examination revealed a slightly elevated total protein of 1.2 g/L, and no leukocytes.

Diagnostic considerations

Our diagnosis of CIDP was based upon:

- Proximal and distal weakness of the limbs being progressive over an eight-week period
- EMG features of a demyelinating polyneuropathy; i.e., nonuniform slowing of motor nerve conduction that is compatible with localized foci of inflammation of peripheral nerves. This is in contrast to CMT1A that is characterized by more

diffuse slowing of nerve conduction (Figures 16.1 and 16.2).
- Increased CSF protein, in combination with otherwise normal laboratory investigations

Follow-up

The patient was treated with IVIg at a dose of 0.4 g/kg body weight for five consecutive days. Muscle strength improved within a few days. However, a few weeks after the first five-day course of IVIg, he deteriorated again. When treated every three weeks with a one-day maintenance dose of 0.4 g/kg body weight, he was able to perform all regular daily activities normally, including his much loved cycling. Over the years, there was some fluctuation in strength of his arms and legs. Especially after the patient had had an infection, weakness sometimes reappeared. In general, however, muscle strength between the IVIg infusions was relatively stable and the patient did not notice a clear deterioration in the days just prior to the next IVIg infusion. Five years later, after a regular attempt (once every 3–4 mo) to reduce the IVIg dosage used in the three-week treatment from 30 g to 20–25 g, it appeared that there was an objective increase in muscle weakness indicating that he still needed maintenance treatment.

General remarks

The clinical and electrophysiological international consensus criteria for CIDP have recently been updated. In CIDP, there is usually progression over a period of at least eight weeks. About 10%–15% of CIDP patients, however, have a relatively rapid progressive course that may initially resemble GBS. If a patient, initially diagnosed with GBS, shows further deterioration or fluctuation of weakness, acute-onset CIDP (A-CIDP) should be considered. Patients initially diagnosed with GBS who have three or more treatment-related fluctuations (TRF; see GBS), or another deterioration eight weeks after onset, are very likely to have A-CIDP (Figure 16.3). Once it is clear that it is CIDP with acute onset, treatment should be the same as for more slowly progressive or relapsing CIDP. Patients with CIDP often have symmetric proximal weakness in addition to distal weakness. CSF total protein is elevated in the majority of patients. Pure

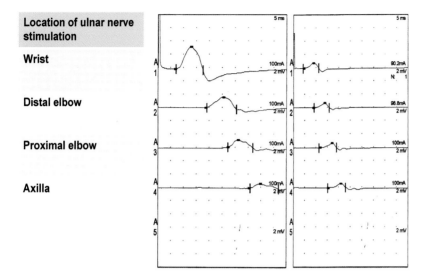

Location of ulnar nerve stimulation
Wrist
Distal elbow
Proximal elbow
Axilla

Figure 16.1. Motor nerve stimulation of the ulnar nerve at different sites; registration of CMAPs at the abductor digiti minimi muscle. Left panel (CIDP): lower amplitudes of the compound muscle action potential (CMAP) at proximal versus distal stimulation indicate conduction block. Reduction of the CMAP at stimulation in the lower arm is 50% compared with stimulation at the wrist. In axonal neuropathy (right panel), the CMAP is too low, irrespective of the site of stimulation.

Stimulus	Demyelinating neuropathy			Axonal neuropathy		
	Latency (ms)	CMAP (mV)	NCV (m/s)	Latency (ms)	CMAP (mV)	NCV (m/s)
Wrist	7.0	3.4	-	4.2	0.9	-
Distal elbow	19.0	1.6	15	9.1	0.8	53
Proximal elbow	27.1	1.1	12	11.2	0.8	48
Axilla	35.7	0.7	17	15.1	0.7	54

Figure 16.2. Motor nerve stimulation of the ulnar nerve at different sites; registration of CMAPs at the abductor digiti minimi muscle. In demyelinating and axonal neuropathy, electrophysiological examination shows differences of DML, MNCVs, and CMAPs. The CIDP patient had increased DMLs, reduced motor NCVs, motor nerve conduction block, and temporal dispersion of the CMAP with proximal versus distal stimulation. The patient with axonal polyneuropathy had normal DMLs and motor NCV, but typically low CMAPs.

sensory CIDP may occur, but is rather rare. It should, therefore, be stressed that the differential diagnosis of sensory neuropathies is wide and includes systemic disorders like Sjögren syndrome and hematological disorders (M-protein); these must be ruled out before starting treatment for sensory CIDP. The best treatment for sensory CIDP has not been studied; it would seem reasonable to assume that treatment with IVIg or steroids could be tried first.

According to the criteria for CIDP, the presence of an IgM M-protein rules out a diagnosis of CIDP, especially when there are antibodies to myelin-associated glycoprotein (MAG). Most patients with an IgM M-protein and anti-MAG antibodies have a mildly progressive sensory ataxic polyneuropathy (Case 20). Finding an IgG M-protein in a patient with CIDP is most probably coincidental, as the incidence increases with aging.

CIDP may improve after treatment with corticosteroids, IVIg, or PE. Most patients need this treatment for a long period of time, ranging from a few months to over 25 years. The primary choice is between steroids and IVIg. If deteriorations with IVIg occur, these can be treated by increasing the IVIg dosage or by shortening the interval between the infusions. Steroids are cheap, but have potentially severe side effects, whereas IVIg treatment is

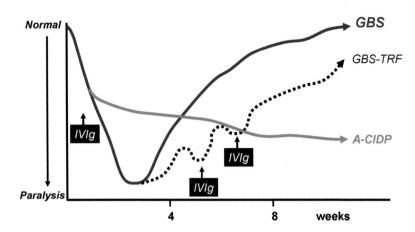

Figure 16.3. Disease course in patients with typical GBS, GBS-TRFs, and acute-onset CIDP (A-CIDP). Patients with A-CIDP are frequently diagnosed with GBS initially. Patients initially diagnosed as GBS with three or more TRFs, or patients who, eight weeks or later after onset, have further deterioration, will likely have CIDP.

expensive, but with a good side-effect profile. PE can be tried if steroids or IVIg appear to fail, but does require special equipment facilities, good vascular access, and is also expensive. If none of these treatments is effective, it would be worthwhile revising the diagnosis before trying one of the other, nonproven, effective immunomodulatory drugs.

Although the diagnosis of CIDP can be difficult, the disease is treatable and most patients have a good prognosis.

Suggested reading

Eftimov F, Winer JB, Vermeulen M, de Haan R, van Schaik IN. Intravenous immunoglobulin for chronic inflammatory demyelinating polyradiculoneuropathy. *Cochrane Database Syst Rev* 2009; CD001797.

European Federation of Neurological Societies/ Peripheral Nerve Society Guideline on management of chronic inflammatory demyelinating polyradiculoneuropathy: report of a joint task force of the European Federation of Neurological Societies and the Peripheral Nerve Society – first rev. *J Peripher Nerv Syst* 2010; **15**: 1–9.

Hughes RA, Mehndiratta MM. Corticosteroids for chronic inflammatory demyelinating polyneuropathy. *Cochrane Database Syst Rev* 2012; CD 002062.

Koller H, Kieseier BC, Jander S, Hartung HP. Chronic inflammatory demyelinating polyneuropathy. *N Engl J Med* 2005; **352**: 1343–1356.

Ruts L, Drenthen J, Jacobs BC, van Doorn PA. Distinguishing acute-onset CIDP from fluctuating Guillain–Barre syndrome: a prospective study. *Neurology* 2010; **74**: 1680–1686.

Multifocal motor neuropathy: a café proprietor with decreased dexterity of the hand and foot drop

Clinical history

A 49-year-old woman experienced increasing diffi-culty with her right hand when taking money out of her purse or fastening buttons. When carving meat she had muscle cramps. Two years later, she noted foot drop after walking some distance. Two neurologists could not decide on a diagnosis. Previous diagnostic tests included a normal MRI of the cervical spine and nerve conduction studies suggesting a carpal tunnel syndrome.

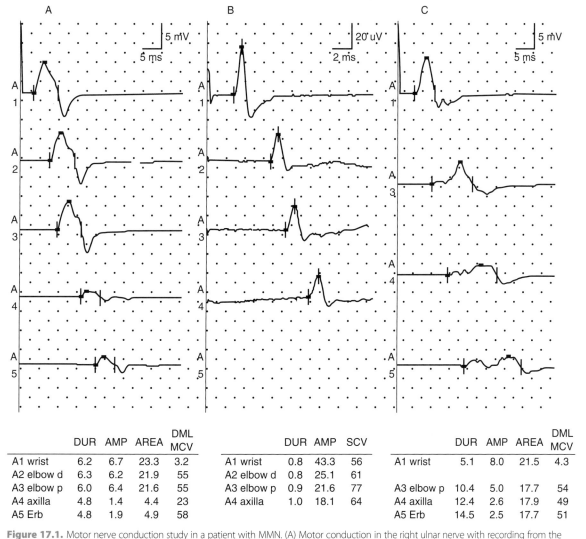

	DUR	AMP	AREA	DML MCV
A1 wrist	6.2	6.7	23.3	3.2
A2 elbow d	6.3	6.2	21.9	55
A3 elbow p	6.0	6.4	21.6	55
A4 axilla	4.8	1.4	4.4	23
A5 Erb	4.8	1.9	4.9	58

	DUR	AMP	SCV
A1 wrist	0.8	43.3	56
A2 elbow d	0.8	25.1	61
A3 elbow p	0.9	21.6	77
A4 axilla	1.0	18.1	64

	DUR	AMP	AREA	DML MCV
A1 wrist	5.1	8.0	21.5	4.3
A3 elbow p	10.4	5.0	17.7	54
A4 axilla	12.4	2.6	17.9	49
A5 Erb	14.5	2.5	17.7	51

Figure 17.1. Motor nerve conduction study in a patient with MMN. (A) Motor conduction in the right ulnar nerve with recording from the muscle abductor digiti minimi. Definite conduction block (CB) and MCV compatible with demyelination were found in the upper arm segment. (B) Sensory conduction in the same nerve, with recording from digiti minimi. No abnormalities were found. (C) Motor conduction in the right median nerve of another patient, with recording from the abductor pollicis brevis muscle. Increased temporal dispersion and probable CB were found in the lower arm segment and probable CB was found in the upper arm segment. elbow d, stimulation 5 cm distally from elbow; elbow p, stimulation 5 cm proximally from elbow; DUR, duration in ms; AMP, amplitude in mV (motor) or μV (sensory); DML, distal motor latency in ms; MCV, motor conduction velocity in m/s; SCV, sensory conduction velocity in m/s. Area in mVms. (From Van Asseldonk JTA, Van den Berg LH, Van den Berg-Vos RM, et al. Demyelination and axonal loss in multifocal motor neuropathy: distribution and relation to weakness. *Brain* 2003; **126**: 186–198, with permission.)

Examination

At the age of 57 years, she was found to have atrophy of the right first dorsal interosseus and thenar muscles and weakness of the following muscles: first dorsal interosseus, MRC grade 4; flexor pollicis, 0; abductor pollicis brevis, 2; opponens, 4; deep and superficial flexors of the second and third fingers, 4. She had weak foot dorsiflexors of the right leg, grade 4. Sensation was normal. Achilles tendon reflexes were absent.

Ancillary investigations

CK activity was normal. A repeat EMG showed conduction block in the tibial nerve and in proximal segments of the right median and ulnar nerves (Figure 17.1). Sensory nerve conduction was normal.

Diagnostic considerations and follow-up

The EMG finding of motor nerve conduction blocks was compatible with the clinical diagnosis of MMN. The late onset, as well as the absence of a history of pressure palsies and of conduction block over nerve compression sites, excluded an alternative diagnosis of HNPP. Following treatment with a five-day course of IVIg (0.4 g/kg), she could again hold a glass of water and muscle cramps disappeared. The foot drop disappeared. She now receives low-frequency maintenance treatment with IVIg.

Table 17.1. Differential diagnosis of multifocal motor neuropathy

Disease/syndrome	Clinical characteristics	EMG and other diagnostic tests
MMN	Distal onset weakness in area of peripheral nerve (2/3 arm) Late skeletal muscular atrophy in affected area Slow progression (months–years)	CB may occur outside clinically affected area CB can be proximal (Erb–axilla segment) MRI and echoscopy of brachial plexus may show thickened nerves CSF not diagnostic
ALS/MND	Distal onset weakness with atrophy UMN signs Rapid progression (weeks–months)	Denervation more generalized No conduction block (CB)
Distal segmental SMA	Distal onset in area of peripheral nerve Slow progression (months–years)	Localized denervation No CB
Motor variant of CIDP	Proximal symmetric weakness and areflexia	Generalized, focal conduction abnormalities: CB, slow conduction, prolonged distal motor latencies and F-waves
MADSAM neuropathy (the Lewis–Sumner syndrome), a variant of CIDP	Distal onset weakness in area of peripheral nerve (2/3 arm) Sensory loss Slow progression (months–years)	Generalized, focal conduction abnormalities: CB, slow conduction, prolonged distal motor latencies and F-waves
Neurogenic thoracic outlet syndrome	Distal onset weakness in C8–T1 muscles Sensory loss in T1 dermatome Usually unilateral Slow progression (months–years)	Reduced or absent medial antebrachial cutaneous SNAP, low ulnar SNAP, denervation C8–T1 muscles Also: prolonged transverse process of seventh rib (X-ray with or without fibrous band on MRI) (Figure 17.3)
HNPP (hereditary neuropathy with liability to pressure palsy)	Acute, remitting peripheral nerve dysfunction from compression (ulnar, peroneal, radial nerves) If severe, neuropathy can become permanent	Slow conduction over compression sites Also: deletion of PMP22 gene
Vasculitic mononeuropathy	Acute motor and sensory dysfunction of peripheral nerve, usually with pain	Acute axonal degeneration can cause pseudoconduction block for up to two weeks, usually shorter
IBM	Slowly progressive weakness of deep finger flexor muscles (months)	No CB of median or ulnar nerves; myopathic with aspecific neurogenic abnormalities

General remarks

MMN was first described some 20 years ago. In essence, MMN is a pure motor neuropathy with slowly progressive weakness of distal limb muscles and motor nerve conduction block (CB) outside nerve compression sites (ulnar groove, fibular head). The prevalence of MMN has been estimated to be 0.6 per 100 000 individuals, and the male to female ratio is 2.7:1. In the Netherlands, the mean age at onset varies between 38 years in men and 45 years in women. Onset is not seen in children or in adults older than 70 years.

In about two-thirds of patients, onset is in the arm, involvement of distal muscles being predominant. The weak muscles belong to the innervation area of a single peripheral nerve. Initially, atrophy is not prominent. Sensation is normal. Reflexes can be absent in affected limbs. Since the recognition of MMN as a specific disorder, diagnostic delay has been reduced, but may still be as long as five years. Nerve conduction studies are obligatory for a diagnosis of MMN (Table 17.1). CSF findings are not diagnostic in MMN. Other laboratory abnormalities include elevation of serum IgM anti-GM1 antibodies in about 40% of cases, and mild elevation of CK activity. Asymmetric high signal intensities on T2 MRI scans of the brachial plexus occur in about 40% of patients (Figure 17.2). These suggest more widespread inflammation of peripheral nerves and have also been demonstrated in CIDP and multifocal acquired demyelinating sensory and motor (MADSAM) neuropathy, the Lewis–Sumner syndrome that is a variant of CIDP (Table 17.1).

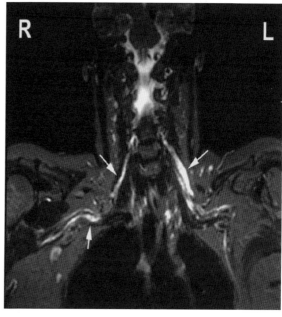

Figure 17.2. Coronal fat-suppressed T2-weighted fast spin-echo MRI scan shows increased focal signal intensities of brachial plexus branches (arrows) in a patient with MMN.

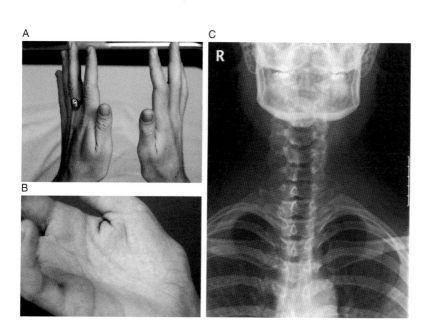

Figure 17.3. Neurogenic thoracic outlet syndrome. (A, B) Atrophy of thenar and first dorsal interosseus muscle of the left hand. (C) X-ray showing prolonged transverse process of right seventh cervical vertebra in another patient.

The cause of MMN is as yet unknown; the hypothesis being that it is an immune dysfunction. Usually, without treatment, severe weakness and atrophy develop, leading to serious functional impairment. When patients are diagnosed at a very late stage, MMN mimics severe PMA with preserved respiration. Patients who experience weakness and functional impairment can be treated, but not cured, with IVIg. Most respond to maintenance therapy. Other immune-modulating therapies have proven unsuccessful.

Suggested reading

Cats EA, van der Pol WL, Piepers S, et al. Correlates of outcome and response to IVIg in 88 patients with multifocal motor neuropathy. *Neurology* 2010; **75**: 818–825.

Van Asseldonk JTH, Franssen H, van den Berg-Vos RM, Wokke JHJ, van den Berg LH. Multifocal motor neuropathy. *Lancet Neurol* 2005; **4**: 309–319.

Vlam L, van der Pol WL, Cats EC, et al. Multifocal motor neuropathy: diagnosis, pathogenesis and treatment strategies. *Nat Rev Neurol* 2011; **8**: 48–58.

CASE 18: Peripheral nerve hyperexcitability syndrome, Morvan's syndrome: an undulating man

Clinical history

For six weeks, a previously healthy 64-year-old man had experienced increasing pain in his back with some referred pain in his hips, knees, and feet. The pain increased when walking. Two or three weeks later he noticed irregular, frequent movements in the muscles of both legs that, after another two weeks, spread toward his arms. Muscle cramps and weakness were not reported. He had symptoms of increased sweating, insomnia, and constipation, but no problem with micturition. His wife noted that he became agitated. He did not have delusions. During this period, he suffered a 12% weight loss with normal appetite. His GP had prescribed benzodiazepines, pregabalin, paracetamol, and morphine with no effect.

He had been a regular cigarette smoker until the age of 50 years. For a number of years he had complained about dull and painful feet and for the past few months had tingling sensations in the fingertips.

Examination

On inspection, profuse undulating myokymia were noticed in all muscles of his limbs and trunk, but not in those of his face or tongue (Video 14). He had mild proximal muscle atrophy of the legs. Muscle tone and strength were normal. He had a stocking-and-glove decrease in pain and tactile sense with absent perception of the tuning fork in the feet. All reflexes were hyperactive, but the Achilles reflexes were absent. Ataxia was not found.

Ancillary investigations

CK activity was 3.5 times ULN, but otherwise analysis of the blood, urine, and CSF was not diagnostic. He had no M-protein. Needle EMG showed myokymic discharges (triplet motor unit potentials) on insertion in all investigated limb muscles. Fasciculation was absent. Motor and sensory nerve conduction studies were normal and signs of axonal degeneration were not found.

After a few weeks, a test of anti-voltage-gated potassium channel (VGKC) antibodies proved positive. Screening for a malignancy, including CT of the chest and abdomen, was negative. No thymoma was detected. A fluorodeoxyglucose–positron emission tomography (FDG–PET) scan revealed generalized lymphadenopathy, but several lymph node biopsies only revealed follicular hyperplasia. A lumbar MRI scan demonstrated severe stenosis at the L4–L5 level.

Diagnostic considerations

Generalized myokymia, combined with autonomic neuropathy, agitation, and sleeping disturbances comprise Morvan's syndrome, one of the peripheral nerve hyperexcitability syndromes. Second, he probably had sensory neuropathy. Finally, he had neurogenic claudication.

Follow-up

He was treated with an intensive course of PE for a period of two months with almost complete disappearance of myokymia, agitation, and hyperhydrosis. He could sleep normally again. The symptoms of sensory neuropathy did not change.

After one year without further treatment, myokymia was observed only in the calves. Renewed screening for a malignancy again proved negative. His walking difficulties had not improved. He declined laminectomy.

General remarks

Spontaneous and continuous muscle over-activity is a sign of generalized peripheral nerve hyperexcitability, or of rippling muscle disease due to caveolinopathy (Case 39). Differentiation can be achieved with electrophysiology. Patients with rippling muscle disease have percussion-induced rapid muscle contractions that are extremely slow (0.6 m/s; i.e., 10 times slower than normal muscle contraction). These contractions are associated with electrical silence on needle EMG. In 1948, Denny-Brown and Foley denominated generalized peripheral nerve hyperexcitability undulating myokymia. Essentially abnormal findings may include myokymic EMG discharges (spontaneous discharges of double, triplet, or multiplet motor units), fasciculations (spontaneous discharges of single motor units), and fibrillations (spontaneous discharges of single muscle fibers). With surface EMG, a maximum of 10 different motor units showing simultaneous myokymic activity can be observed. Pseudomyotonia, persisting muscle contraction caused by continuous firing of motor units, is observed in a large number of patients. Some patients with myokymia also have peripheral sensory neuropathy. Nerve conduction studies may be normal, suggesting small nerve fiber neuropathy, as in the presented case.

Myokymia can be so profuse that the patient appears to undulate with continuous waves under the skin (Video 14). Pseudomyotonia and myokymia form the hallmark of Isaac's syndrome, neuromyotonia. Autonomic signs are less prevalent and CNS signs

are absent in neuromyotonia, but the boundary with Morvan's syndrome has not yet been well defined.

Morvan's syndrome consists of myokymia, dysautonomia, and CNS manifestations: insomnia, tonic-clonic seizures, faciobrachial dystonic seizures, mood change, visual hallucinations, and delusions. Features of dysautonomia may include hyperhidrosis, constipation, tachycardia, orthostatic hypotension, and QT interval prolongation. Males are affected predominantly.

Many patients with peripheral nerve hyperexcitability syndrome have muscle cramps and stiffness. Some experience weakness. Exercise usually triggers myokymia. Some patients have associated myasthenia gravis, usually with anti-AChR antibodies. Up to a third of patients with Morvan's syndrome have a thymoma. CK activity is raised in about half of the patients.

Both Morvan's syndrome and Isaac's syndrome are autoimmune diseases that occur with and without neoplasms. The causative role of anti-VGKC antibodies has been recognized recently. They are directed against VGKCs at terminal nerve endings at the neuromuscular junction, and–in Morvan's syndrome–at neuronal and glial VGKCs. In essence, these peripheral nerve hyperexcitability syndromes are autoimmune disorders with antibodies acting against extracellular antigens, whereas in subacute sensory paraneoplastic neuropathy (Case 22), antineuronal antibodies are directed against intracellular antigens. The implication of this notion is that immunotherapy can be effective. With PE (Video 14), IVIg, or immunosuppression with steroids and azathioprine, recovery can be achieved. Relapses may occur.

Suggested reading

Denny-Brown D, Foley DM. Myokymia and the benign fasciculation or muscular cramps. *Trans Assoc Am Physicians* 1948; **61**: 88–96.

Hart IK, Maddison P. Newsom-Davis J, Vincent A, Mills K. Phenotypic variants of peripheral nerve hyperexcitability. *Brain* 2002; **125**: 1887–1895.

Irani SR, Pettingill P, Kleopa K, et al. Morvan syndrome: clinical and serological observations in 29 cases. *Ann Neurol* 2012; **72**: 241–245.

Vasculitic neuropathy: a man with painful bilateral foot drop and tingling hands

Clinical history

A 53-year-old man complained of severe pain in his back and legs for the past four months. He developed drop feet (starting on the left side) during that period, and as a consequence, stumbled easily. In addition, he noticed progressive numbness of his lower legs and painful feet. His arms and especially his hands were very sensitive when tapped. He had no further symptoms and his medical history was not informative. He did not recall a tick bite or erythema migrans, or any pulmonary abnormality.

Examination

Walking was impaired due to bilateral foot drop. Cranial nerves were normal. He had no atrophy or sensory disturbances of the arms or hands. There appeared to be minor atrophy of the muscles of the upper legs. He was, however, unable to stand on his heels and could barely stand on his toes. Several muscle groups were paretic: predominantly the hamstrings, peronei, anterior and posterior tibial muscles, and the triceps surae, MRC grade 4. Pain, touch, and vibration senses were impaired in the feet. Achilles tendon reflexes were absent. Radicular provocation tests were negative. Clinical examination of the skin revealed signs suggestive of vasculitis (Figure 19.1).

Ancillary investigations

C-reactive protein (CRP) was 11 (<10); the number of eosinophilic granulocytes was slightly raised. Antibodies ANA were 1:160 (normally: negative), and ANCA, SS-A,

and SS-B were negative. He had no M-protein; liver enzymes and creatinine levels were normal. Serological testing for lues and Lyme disease proved negative. Concentric needle analysis showed denervation potentials in muscles innervated by L5 and S1 nerve roots. Motor nerve action potentials of the tibial and peroneal nerves were decreased, compatible with axonal degeneration. Sural nerve action potentials were absent. Analysis of motor conduction of arm nerves showed no signs of demyelination. CSF analysis revealed a slightly elevated protein content, 0.5 g/L (<0.45), and mild pleocytosis of 8×10^6 lymphocytes/L (<4). Repeat lumbar puncture produced similar results, again with no malignant cells.

A lumbar spine MRI scan was normal. The sural nerve biopsy showed clear signs of vasculitis with fibrinoid necrosis of the vascular wall (Figure 19.2).

Follow-up

The patient was diagnosed with vasculitis, predominantly or only in the peripheral nervous system. He was treated with prednisone, 60 mg/day. Pain decreased and sensory abnormalities improved. Weakness did not progress further and tended to improve over the next few months. Muscle strength eventually improved over a period of eight months to nearly normal.

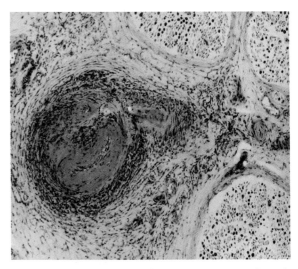

Figure 19.2. Sural nerve biopsy showing necrotizing vasculitis with fibrinoid necrosis of the vascular wall with inflammatory cell infiltrate. (Hematoxylin-and-eosin staining, x150).

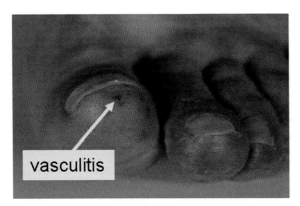

vasculitis

Figure 19.1. Skin lesions suggestive of vasculitis.

General remarks

Most patients with vasculitis have systemic features, but some have only neurological manifestations. In the latter group, low titers of ANA and minor elevated levels of CRP or erythrocyte sedimentation rate (ESR) can be found. A nonsystemic vasculitic neuropathy is a rare disease that usually has a subacute onset with progressive sensory or sensorimotor deficits. Asymmetry, pain, and weakness are key features. As shown in this case, not all patients with vasculitis have clear asymmetric features over time; some may present with painful symmetric involvement resembling a polyneuropathy.

The diagnosis of nonsystemic vasculitis can only be made by excluding other causes; for example, by the absence of clinical signs of systemic vasculitis, and the absence of clearly positive ANA, ANCA, or SS-A/SS-B. In addition, the vasculitis (not only a perivascular infiltrate) has to be demonstrated in a nerve or a combined nerve and muscle biopsy.

Corticosteroids are the mainstay of treatment for systemic vasculitis, but what the best treatment is for nonsystemic vasculitis has not yet been established. Nor is it known whether or which type of immunosuppressive treatment (cytotoxic drugs) needs to be administered in addition to steroids, or can function as an alternative for steroids – especially in patients with a relative contraindication for long-term, high-dose steroids.

The prognosis varies for improvement of the neuropathy. In patients with systemic vasculitis, the disease course may be very severe and even lethal. In nonsystemic vasculitis, the progression is generally slower than in systemic vasculitis and the prognosis better. These patients have, therefore, a better prognosis, but steroid treatment may be required for a long period of time. Long-term follow-up studies show that most patients can walk without assistance and are independent as far as activities of daily living are concerned.

Suggested reading

Collins MP, Dyck PJ, Gronseth GS, et al. Peripheral Nerve Society Guideline on the classification, diagnosis, investigation, and immunosuppressive therapy of nonsystemic vasculitic neuropathy: executive summary. *J Peripher Nerv Syst* 2010; **15**: 176–184.

Schaublin GA, Michet CL, Dyck PJ, Burns TM. An update in the classification and the treatment of vasculitis neuropathy. *Lancet Neurol* 2005; **4**: 853–865.

Vrancken AF, Hughes RA, Said G, Wokke JH, Notermans NC. Immunosuppressive treatment for non-systemic vasculitic neuropathy. *Cochrane Database Syst Rev* 2007; CD006050.

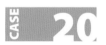

Neuropathy and ataxia caused by immunoglobulin-M gammopathy: a 79-year-old woman with nocturnal headaches who could no longer play bridge

Clinical history

From the age of 53 years, this lady had been suffering from severe nocturnal headaches. At age 68 years, a diagnosis of hypnic headache was made. She was treated accordingly with lithium carbonate. At that time, results of the neurological examination were normal. Aged 69 years of age, the headaches subsided but she developed severe tremor of both hands that hindered her in holding her cards, and drinking a glass of wine. She could no longer walk steadily carrying a tray of teacups. A relationship with lithium carbonate was suggested, but she did not dare stop taking the drug because of the beneficial effect on her headaches. When 73 years old, she complained of a sensation of numbness under both feet. The tremor of the hands had increased.

Examination

She had a stocking-and-glove sensory loss with a marked postural and kinetic tremor of both arms (Video 15). Below the hips she could not feel the vibration of the tuning fork. Kinesthesia of the toes was impaired and she had mild rombergism. Tandem walking was not possible. She had no weakness. Reflexes were absent in the legs.

71

Ancillary investigations

Routine analysis of the blood and vitamin B12, B6, and E concentrations were normal. She had a monoclonal IgM kappa protein that could not be quantified. Total IgM concentration was 2.2 (<2.3) g/L. Using erythrocyte-linked immunosorbent assay (ELISA) serum IgM anti-MAG, antibodies were demonstrated. Nerve conduction studies showed markedly increased distal motor latencies and less pronounced slowing of motor nerve conduction in the median and ulnar nerves in forearm segments (40–43 m/s). SNAP amplitudes were reduced. Bone marrow analysis showed 15%–20% IgM and kappa light chain positive B lymphocytes (normally absent).

Diagnostic considerations and follow-up

The hematologist diagnosed lymphocytic plasmacytoma and IgM kappa monoclonal gammopathy. Because of the low malignancy grade and absence of systemic B-symptoms – fever >38°C, bouts of sweating especially at night, and weight loss >10% over six months – treatment was not indicated. During a five-year follow-up, her hematological condition remained stable.

The sensory ataxic, axonal neuropathy bothered her more and more with walking (Video 15). The dosage of lithium carbonate was decreased as the drug can cause increased tremor. Two years after the diagnosis of the neuropathy, she was treated with rituximab without clinical effect; nor was there a change in serum IgM. Seven years after diagnosis, she had become so unstable that she needed a rollator.

General remarks

Monoclonal gammopathy of undetermined significance (MGUS) is by definition a premalignant, asymptomatic disorder characterized by:

- Monoclonal cell proliferation in bone marrow
- No end-organ damage
- Absence of B-cell proliferative disorder

If MGUS is detected, patients must be monitored for progressive hematological disease – myeloma (11% life-long risk), macroglobulinemia (IgM), lymphoproliferative disorders, and light chain amyloidosis – which can occur throughout life. Osteoporosis, vertebral column fractures, and peripheral neuropathy are also associated with MGUS. The occurrence of MGUS (IgG: IgM ~ 4.5:1) increases with age from 0.5% to 2% in persons aged 50–59 years, to 4.0%–8.0% in those over 80 years old (Figure 20.1).

MGUS is a frequent finding in patients with a neuropathy. Neuropathies, whatever the cause, are frequent in individuals aged over 50 years. Consequently, MGUS, whether of the IgG or IgM type, is most probably coincidental in mild chronic axonal neuropathy with no established cause. A causal relationship with CIDP that fulfils electrophysiological and clinical criteria for CIDP is, for the same reason, unlikely. However, in patients with a M-protein and prevailing motor symptoms and signs, CIDP must be excluded by nerve conduction studies of motor nerves.

In contrast, most IgM–MGUS-associated neuropathies are characterized by distal, symmetric

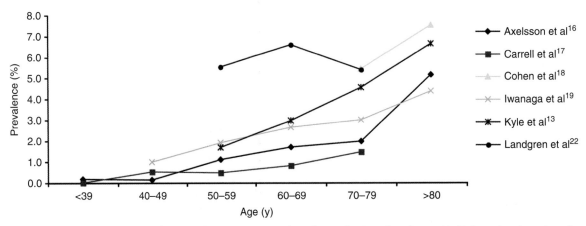

Figure 20.1. Increasing incidence of MGUS with aging. A meta-analysis of 14 studies. Not all studies provided information about class of gammopathy. Some patients had biclonal or multoclonal spikes. (From Wadhera RK, Rajkumar SV. Prevalence of monoclonal gammopathy of undetermined significance: a systematic review. *Mayo Clin Proc* 2010; **85**: 933–942, with permission. References (superscripts) as per source).

sensorimotor and ataxic features. The latter include postural and kinetic tremor and rombergism.

Diagnosis of IgM–MGUS-associated neuropathy is usually reached after a median delay of over three years after the first manifestations. About 50% of patients with IgM–MGUS have circulating anti-MAG antibodies. These have been found to be associated more frequently with kappa chains compared to lambda light chains. The diagnostic value of antibodies to other neural antigens, including gangliosides, is uncertain.

Nerve conduction studies show signs of demyelination in most patients, with pure axonal features in a minority.

Evidence for a causal relationship between IgM and neuropathy stems from pathological and experimental studies. First, IgM deposits can be demonstrated on peripheral nerve myelin sheaths in sural nerve biopsies. Second, passive transfer of IgM from patients may induce demyelination and neuropathy in experimental animals, nerve biopsies showing widening of myelin lamellae. Third, antibodies react with the HNK-1 epitope of MAG that, interestingly, also happens to be present on the PMP22 protein. This latter finding and the observation of slowing of nerve conduction at pressure sites in patients suggest that anti-MAG neuropathy due to acquired loss of PMP22 function resembles hereditary liability to pressure palsy neuropathy.

Follow-up analysis showed that demyelination, older age at onset, and absence of anti-MAG antibodies are associated with a poorer outcome (Figure 20.2).

Evidence-based treatment strategies for IgM–MGUS-associated neuropathies are lacking. Therapies that have been evaluated include IVIg, PE, corticosteroids, interferon-alpha, chlorambucil, and fludarabine. In one trial, combined therapy of intermittent cyclophosphamide and prednisone had an effect on secondary, but not primary outcome measures. A similar result, with fewer side effects, was observed in a trial with the humanized antibody against the CD20 antigen, rituximab. Some patients clearly benefitted. The effect is usually noticed after three to six months and may last for two to three years. A systematic review, however, concluded that the evidence for benefit from rituximab is of very low quality.

First-choice drugs for treatment of tremor – similar to treatment of essential tremor – are propranolol and primidone.

Furthermore, CANOMAD syndrome is a rare chronic ataxic neuropathy with ophthalmoplegia, M-protein, cold agglutinins, and disialosyl antibodies. Progression in CANOMAD syndrome is usually more rapid compared to IgM–MGUS neuropathy with anti-MAG antibodies. Patients with CANOMAD syndrome may respond to IVIg and to rituximab treatment.

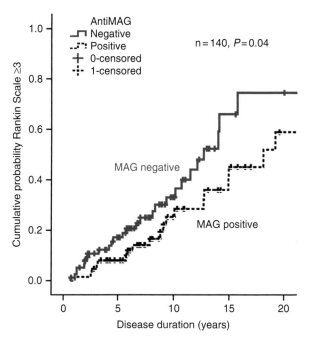

Figure 20.2. Risk of development of modified Rankin Scale ≥3 in a cohort of 140 patients with polyneuropathy associated with immunoglobulin-M monoclonal gammopathy. (From Niermeijer JMF, Fischer K, Eurelings M, et al. Prognosis of polyneuropathy due to IgM monoclonal gammopathy. *Neurology* 2010; **74**: 406–412, with permission.)

Suggested reading

Faber CG, Notermans NC, Wokke JH, Franssen H. Entrapment in anti-myelin-associated glycoprotein neuropathy. *J Neurol* 2009; **256**: 620–624.

Joint Task Force of the EFNS and the PNS. European Federation of Neurological Societies/Peripheral Nerve Society Guideline on management of paraproteinemic demyelinating neuropathies. Report of a Joint Task Force of the European Federation of Neurological Societies and the Peripheral Nerve Society – first rev. *J Peripher Nerv Syst* 2010; **15**: 185–195.

Lunn MP, Nobile-Orazio E. Immunotherapy for IgM anti-myelin-associated glycoprotein paraprotein-associated peripheral neuropathies. *Cochrane Database Syst Rev* 2012; **5**: CD002827.

Niermeijer JMF, Eurelings M. Lokhorst HL, et al. Rituximab for polyneuropathy with IgM monzoclonal gammopathy. *J Neurol Neurosurg Psychiatry* 2009; **80**: 1036–1039.

Niermeijer JMF, Fischer K, Eurelings M, et al. Prognosis of polyneuropathy due to IgM monoclonal gammopathy. *Neurology* 2010; **74**: 406–412.

Nobile-Orazio E. Update on neuropathies associated with monoclonal gammopathy of undetermined significance (2008–2010). *J Peripher Nerv Syst* 2010; **15**: 302–306.

Patwa HS, Chaudhry V, Katzberg H, et al. Evidence-based guideline: intravenous immunoglobulin in the treatment of neuromuscular disorders: report of the therapeutics and technology assessment subcommittees of the American Academy of Neurology. *Neurology* 2012; **78**: 1009–1015.

Wadhera RK, Rajkumar SV. Prevalence of monoclonal gammopathy of undetermined significance: a systematic review. *Mayo Clin Proc* 2010; **85**: 933–942.

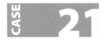

Polyneuropathy, organomegaly, endocrine manifestations, monoclonal protein, and skin changes, POEMS: a man with weight loss, progressive weakness, and burning pain in the legs

CASE 21

Clinical history

A 35-year-old man noticed progressive pain, tingling feelings, and numbness of his legs that became incapacitating over a six-month period. He developed progressive weakness of both feet, which made it difficult to walk and impossible to climb stairs without using his arms. Over the past four months, he had spontaneously lost 15 kg of weight and complained about night sweats and fatigue. For years he had smoked 40 cigarettes per day.

Examination

A general examination revealed no overt abnormalities with the exception of some bluish discoloration of his feet. He had weakness of the intrinsic hand muscles, MRC grade 4–5, and his grasp force had clearly decreased. His upper legs were symmetrically paretic (MRC grade 4). He had weakness and mild atrophy of the lower legs, MRC grade 3–4 (Figure 21.1). There was diminished sensation for pain and touch in the hands and distal to the knees.

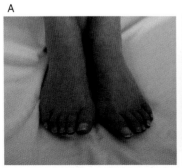
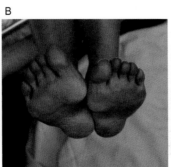
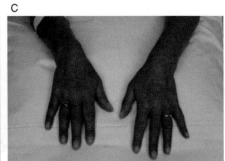

Figure 21.1. (A–C) Mild Ratnaud phenomenon in a 47-year-old woman with POEMS. Atrophy of the abductor hallucis muscles (A, B).

Vibration sense was impaired in the hands and feet. There was generalized areflexia.

Ancillary investigations

Routine blood examination showed no abnormalities but a slightly elevated glucose level and an IgG lambda monoclonal spike (6 g/L). IgM was slightly increased (maximum 6 g/L); there was no IgM paraprotein. TSH was normal. Nerve conduction studies revealed a severe motor and sensory demyelinating polyneuropathy. X-ray analysis of the skeleton showed a sclerotic lesion in the ramus superior of the left pubic bone (Figure 21.2). CT scans of the thorax and abdomen were performed later and revealed an enlarged liver and spleen. The results of full hematological screening, including the total IgG level, were otherwise normal.

Diagnostic considerations

Initially the patient was diagnosed with a demyelinating polyneuropathy that was clinically compatible with CIDP. Nerve conduction studies fulfilled criteria for CIDP. The presence of an IgG monoclonal gammopathy worried us, especially in combination with his young age and weight loss. Because of the relative rapidity with which weakness progressed, we decided to initiate steroid treatment, and he clearly improved. As we kept the possibility of a hematological malignancy in mind, an extended systemic survey was performed that showed an enlarged liver and spleen. The combination of a demyelinating polyneuropathy, enlarged liver and spleen, elevated glucose, and the presence of a M-protein were compatible with the

diagnosis of POEMS. Symptoms of weight loss and night sweats can occur in patients with a hematological malignancy.

Follow-up

The patient was treated with melphalan and prednisone. The sclerotic bone lesion was treated with local radiation. He made a very good recovery. Signs and symptoms of polyneuropathy almost completely disappeared within a year. The follow-up period now exceeds 10 years; he only has a mild foot drop and minor distal sensory disturbances of the feet. Hematological controls did not reveal a further rise of the serum IgG-lambda M-protein.

General remarks

POEMS is a plasma-proliferative disorder. The diagnosis should be considered by neurologists if a patient with a chronic polyneuropathy, that may resemble CIDP, has an M-protein and systemic symptoms.

Not all patients demonstrate all five symptoms encrypted into the acronym POEMS. Some may also have nephropathy or pachymeningitis.

Establishing a diagnosis of POEMS can be difficult, resulting in a diagnostic delay in most patients. Recently, it was shown that serum levels of vascular endothelial growth factor (VEGF) are elevated abnormally, and this is now considered to be one of the major criteria for making the diagnosis. Patients with POEMS can be treated with radiotherapy (if there is a sclerotic bone lesion), immunomudulatory drugs with or without chemotherapy, and bone marrow transplantation. It is not clear what the best treatment is; a risk-adapted approach to therapy is required. Combined therapy with melphalan and dexamethasone seems promising. Severity of the clinical phenotype, age, and general condition of the patient are factors that must be considered when deciding whether to administer cytostatic drugs.

Suggested reading

Dispenzieri A. POEMS syndrome: 2011 update on diagnosis, risk-stratification, and management. *Am J Hematol* 2011; **86**: 591–601.

Kuwabara S, Dispenzieri A, Arimura K, Misawa S. Treatment for POEMS (polyneuropathy, organomegaly, endocrinopathy, M-protein, and skin changes) syndrome. *Cochrane Database Syst Rev* 2008; CD006828.

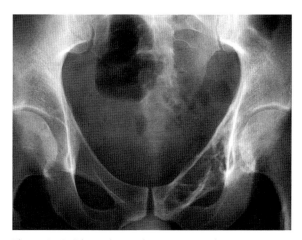

Figure 21.2. Sclerotic lesion, plasmacytoma, in the ramus superior of the left pubic bone.

Li J, Zhang W, Li J, et al. Combination of melphalan and dexamethasone for patients with newly diagnosed POEMS syndrome. *Blood* 2011; **117**: 6445–6449.

Scarlato M, Previtali SC. POEMS syndrome: the matter-of-fact approach. *Curr Opin Neurol* 2011; **24**: 491–496.

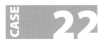

CASE 22

Subacute sensory paraneoplastic neuropathy and ganglionopathy: an elderly lady with "plastic" feet

Clinical history

A 73-year-old woman suddenly noticed pain in her lower and upper right leg and left foot. After a few weeks of physical therapy, she gradually developed tingling in her feet and a "plastic" sensation in the soles. A few weeks later, her feet had become completely numb and painful tingling had developed in her hands and around her left knee. Because of the tingling in her hands, she could barely use a knife and fork. Walking became difficult due to the dull feelings in her legs. Various drugs for painful neuropathy failed to help.

For years she had smoked two packs of cigarettes a week. A total of 50 pack–years was estimated.

Examination

The cranial nerves were normal. Pain and tactile sense were impaired in her hands and absent in the feet distally from just above the ankles. Vibration and position sense appeared normal, but she demonstrated sensory ataxia on the knee–heel test. There was minor bilateral weakness of the extensor hallucis longus muscles. Knee tendon reflexes were low; Achilles tendon reflexes were absent. Walking was difficult and broad-based. While standing with the eyes closed, she had impressive rombergism.

Ancillary investigations

Routine laboratory analysis of the blood did not reveal any abnormalities. Motor and sensory conduction velocities were normal, but SNAP amplitudes were decreased.

A CT scan of the thorax revealed a tumor in her right lung. Pathological examination demonstrated a small-cell lung carcinoma (SCLC). CSF analysis showed a mononuclear pleocytosis of 14×10^6 cells (Normal < 4) and a protein level of 0.64 g/L. There were no tumor cells. Serum anti-Hu antibodies were positive.

Diagnostic considerations and follow-up

She was diagnosed with subacute sensory paraneoplastic neuropathy and ganglionopathy (neuronopathy) and received systemic chemotherapy and chest radiotherapy. She reached remission of SCLC and reported fewer sensory disturbances. The neurological examination did not, however, change.

General remarks

Sensory neuronopathies, ganglionopathies, are a specific subgroup of peripheral neuropathies characterized by primary and selective dorsal root ganglion (DRG) neuronal destruction. Inflammatory damage to DRG neurons and their projections often results in a multifocal pattern of sensory deficits. This contrasts with the usual length-dependent pattern found in most polyneuropathies. By far the most common associated malignancy is SCLC.

The onset can be asymmetric, distal, or proximal with painful paresthesias or dysesthesias. Although onset generally is subacute with progression over months, progression over days to weeks is no exception. A sensory neuronopathy usually predates detection of a malignancy, but can occur at any point during the course of cancer, even during or after chemotherapy, or after radiation. Older reports, indicating a delay of more than two years between onset of neuropathy and detection of SCLC, date from the period before standard screening with high-quality CT imaging.

Although all sensory modalities can be involved, proprioceptive loss is generally prominent with sensory ataxia that can sometimes lead to pseudoathetosis. Numbness may occur over time. Weakness may develop, but this makes an association with SCLC less likely. One should bear in mind that profound loss of proprioception can seriously hamper

Table 22.1. Causes of sensory ataxic neuronopathies and neuropathies

- Immune-mediated paraneoplastic with anti-Hu (or anti-CV2/CRMP-5) antibodies
- Immune-mediated due to Sjögren syndrome
- Sensory variant of CIDP
- IgM monoclonal gammopathy
- Miller–Fisher syndrome
- Pyridoxine (vitamin B6) deficiency or intoxication
- Use of cis-platin or taxol (dose-dependent)
- Polymerase gamma (POLG1) mutation – compound heterozygosity: sensory ataxic neuropathy with dysarthria and ophthalmoparesis (SANDO). Onset can be in the eighth decade
- Kennedy disease
- SCA17
- Idiopathic

(See also Table 7 of Introduction.)

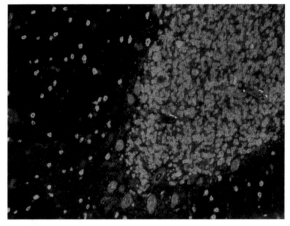

Figure 22.1. Immunofluoresence binding of anti-Hu antibodies to dorsal root ganglion cells (courtesy Professor P.A.E. Sillevis Smitt).

movement as there is no feedback (of movements). There may be associated autonomic symptoms. A usual consequence of proprioceptive sensory loss is the disappearance of deep tendon reflexes.

These features are, however, not specific for this disease. Sensory neuronopathies and neuropathies can have many causes (Table 22.1). Clinical predominant sensory ataxic neuropathy can also be seen in atypical cases of CIDP – or during the course of CIDP. CIDP patients have decreased motor nerve conduction, a feature not characteristic of sensory neuronopathies. Patients with neuropathy associated with IgM monoclonal gammopathy have a more or less stocking-and-glove type of neuropathy with an indolent disease course.

A model, based on the initial clinical and electrophysiological work-up, has been created that can help to diagnose sensory neuronopathy. The presence of sensory ataxia, asymmetric distribution, sensory loss not only in the legs, and the presence of sensory and absence of motor nerve conduction abnormalities, and especially the presence of serum anti-Hu/ANNA-1 (antinuclear antibody) antibodies favor the diagnosis of paraneoplastic sensory neuronopathy.

If the cause cannot be identified easily, one should look for SCLC (smoking history) or Sjögren syndrome. In order to screen for SCLC, a CT scan of the thorax is recommended. If negative, FDG–PET can be indicated. Other tumors (neuroblastoma, breast, prostate and ovarian carcinoma, and thymoma) are far less frequently associated with sensory neuronopathy.

SNAPs may be absent or reduced, but can be normal. Motor nerve conduction studies are mostly normal. The serum should be evaluated, especially for the presence of anti-Hu/ANNA-1 (and VC2/CRMP-5) antibodies. Using immunofluoresence binding of these antibodies to DRG cells can be demonstrated (Figure 22.1). CSF frequently shows a minor rise in mononuclear cells and increased protein content. CSF abnormalities and acute or subacute onset argue strongly for a paraneoplastic origin.

The prognosis depends upon the type of tumor. There is no proven effective treatment for a tumor-related sensory neuronopathy. If the neuropathy precedes the direct symptoms of the tumor, the prognosis may be better because of early detection and treatment of the malignancy.

Suggested reading

Camdessanché JP, Joussereand G, Ferraud K, et al. The pattern and diagnostic criteria of sensory neuronopathy: a case-control study. *Brain* 2009; **132**: 1723–1733.

Koike H, Tanaka F, Sobue G. Paraneoplastic neuropathy: wide-range clinicopathological manifestations. *Curr Opin Neurol* 2011; **24**: 504–510.

Titulaer MJ, Soffietti R, Dalmau J, et al. Screening for tumors in paraneoplastic syndromes: a report of an EFNS task force. *Eur J Neurol* 2011; **18**: 19–27.

Neurolymphomatosis: a sailor with suspected polymyalgia rheumatica, weight loss, and walking difficulties

Clinical history

Over a period of six months, a 70-year-old man who had always been very strong and had worked as a shipmate until the age of 60 years, experienced severe pain in the shoulder and later in the hip regions. A rheumatologist diagnosed polymyalgia rheumatica. Prednisone caused the pain to abate. In the subsequent six months, he complained of numbness that started in both feet and crept upward to his knees, and also of numb hands. Simultaneously, he experienced weakness of the legs. He could no longer walk upstairs or cope with his rollator. He had a good appetite, but nevertheless lost 20 kg of weight. Periods of fever and night sweats were absent. Being a strict Calvinist, he only drank two glasses of jenever (Dutch gin) on Sundays.

Examination

He had marked symmetric atrophy with MRC grade 4 weakness of intrinsic hand and arm muscles (Figure 23.1). The power in his deltoid muscles was MRC grade 4–5 with normal wrist and finger flexor strength. Leg weakness was asymmetric, more pronounced proximally. Strength of his left hip and knee flexors was MRC grade 3. He had a stocking-and-glove loss of sensation with areflexia. He could not feel the vibration of the tuning fork at the knees.

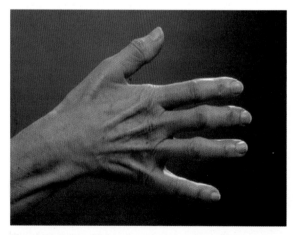

Figure 23.1. Atrophic hand muscles in a patient with neurolymphomatosis. Because of weakness of the intrinsic muscles, the extended fingers cannot be kept together.

Ancillary investigations

All known causes for axonal neuropathy were excluded by appropriate tests. ESR, CRP, and CK activity were normal. Electrophysiological assessment suggested axonal sensory and motor neuropathy. No antibodies to *Treponema pallidum*, *Borrelia burgdorferi*, and *Varicella zoster* virus were found; other antimicrobial tests were also negative. There was no evidence of sarcoidosis. The CSF protein level was 2.3 g/L (< 0.4 g/L) with 2.10 g/L mononuclear cells (< 4/L). Immunophenotyping of the CSF cells showed a monoclonal CD19 positive B-cell population with a kappa/lamda ratio of 98:2, suggesting infiltration by a B-cell lymphoma. Bone marrow analysis, CT imaging of the neck, chest, and abdomen, a FDG–PET scan, and ophthalmological examination were normal. Amyloid deposits and intravascular lymphoma cells were absent from a sural nerve biopsy. The biopsy showed severe axonal degeneration with 3694 myelinated nerve fibers/mm^2 (normal>6695); only small nerve fibers were present.

An MRI scan of the spine showed diffusely thickened and contrast-enhancing cauda equina roots (Figure 23.2). At the cervical level, discrete abnormalities were observed.

Diagnostic considerations and follow-up

He was diagnosed with neurolymphomatosis. He responded well to systemic chemotherapy, including cytarabine and vincristine with normalization of CSF; during a two-year follow-up period his neurological function stabilized. A repeat MRI of the spine was normal.

General remarks

Infiltration of the intraspinal nerve roots by lymphoma cells caused severe distal Wallerian degeneration of peripheral nerves in this patient. This disease is called neurolymphomatosis— primary CNS lymphoma. Retrospectively, the initial symptoms, shoulder pain, could have been a first manifestation of spinal radicular involvement. On referral and prior to diagnosis, he had a one-year history of severe muscle atrophy and areflexia resulting from axonal degeneration. A differential diagnosis of CIDP was considered but rejected after neurophysiological testing. In this patient, CSF analysis and MRI led to the diagnosis of neurolymphomatosis. Diagnostic considerations in progressive multiple mononeuropathies and/or radiculopathies are presented in Table 23.1.

Lymphoma and neuropathy are frequently associated, the usual cause being treatment with vincristine. A second but rare explanation is paraneoplastic neuropathy. Probably even more rare are neurolymphomatosis and intravascular, angiotrophic lymphoma.

Table 23.1. Differential diagnosis of progressive multiple mononeuropathies and/or radiculopathies

- Neuroborreliosis
- Meningitis tuberculosa
- Neurosarcoidosis
- Systemic and nonsystemic vasculitis
- Cryoglobulinemia and primary amyloidosis–both associated with M-protein
- Paraneoplastic neuropathy
- Leptomeningeal carcinomatosis, lymphomatosis
- Meningeal localization of myeloma
- MADSAM, a variant of CIDP

Neurolymphomatosis is defined as nerve infiltration by neoplastic cells in the setting of a known or unknown hematological malignancy, usually B-cell non-Hodgkin lymphoma or acute lymphoblastic leukemia. Lymphoma cells frequently invade the endoneurium. These infiltrating cells do not cause fibrinoid necrosis of the vessel as in vasculitis.

About one-quarter of patients have primary neurolymphomatosis with peripheral or cranial nerve root or plexus dysfunction, or combinations as the first manifestation. Primary neurolymphomatosis is a diagnosis by exclusion. MRI and PET scans may help to detect and localize nerves that are infiltrated by lymphoma cells. Diffuse or nodular thickening of nerves is a common MRI finding. Demonstration of lymphoma cells in CSF or affected nerves warrants aggressive treatment with methotrexate, cytarabin, or both. If successful, stabilization and prolonged survival can be achieved but one cannot expect much improvement in the axonal neuropathy. Radiotherapy at symptomatic sites may be indicated for relief of neuropathic pain.

Suggested reading
Briani C, Vitaliani R, Grisold W, et al. Spectrum of paraneoplastic disease associated with lymphoma. *Neurology* 2011; **76**: 705–710.

A

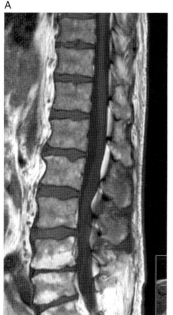

B

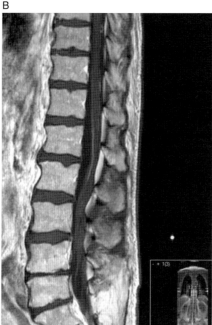

C

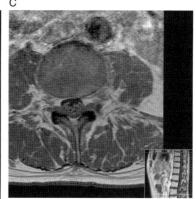

Figure 23.2. T1-weighted MRI scan of the spine showing diffusely thickened (A) and contrast-enhancing cauda equina roots (B, C).

Grisariu S, Avni B, Batchelor TT, et al.
Neurolymphomatosis: an International Primary CNS
Collaborative Group report. *Blood* 2010; **115**: 5005–5011.

Kelly JJ, Karcher DS. Lymphoma and peripheral
neuropathy: a clinical review. *Muscle Nerve* 2005;
31: 301–313.

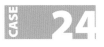

Diabetic polyneuropathy: a woman with diabetes mellitus and slowly progressive painful tingling in her feet

Clinical history

A 52-year-old-woman had had type 2 diabetes mellitus for 10 years. For some time she had had symptoms of slowly progressive tingling in the feet and a feeling of walking on cotton wool.

Over the past few years, the tingling in her feet had become painful and the sensory level had progressed up to the level of her knees. During the previous six months she had had several small wounds on her feet. She noticed some difficulty when walking in the dark, especially on uneven ground. She had no problems with her hands or fingers, and had no clear symptoms of autonomic failure. She has been treated with oral antidiabetics for several years but eventually required insulin. Because of the pain in her feet she often needed paracetamol, which gave her some relief.

Examination

She has minor distal sensory disturbances of the fingers, with a two-point discrimination of 7 mm (≤5 mm, static testing). Recently, the two-point discrimination was reassessed using an esthesiometer giving normative age-related values. Biceps and triceps reflexes were low. There was no weakness. Examination of the legs showed sensory disturbances for pain and touch, up to the level of her knees. Vibration sense was absent distally from the knees. Knee tendon reflexes were decreased and Achilles tendon reflexes were absent. Walking was normal.

Ancillary investigations

Fasting glucose was 8 mmol/L (<6.0). There were no other abnormalities on routine blood examination. EMG showed signs of an axonal polyneuropathy.

Diagnostic considerations and follow-up

The patient had symptoms and signs of a polyneuropathy due to diabetes mellitus. Treatment of pain with low dose amitriptyline was initiated. As this proved ineffective and as she complained of side effects, pregabalin was prescribed. She was also given information on how to prevent development of a diabetic foot.

General remarks

Diabetes mellitus is the most frequent cause of polyneuropathy. Roughly one in 10 people has or will get diabetes (incidence varies between countries and among populations). As about half the patients with diabetes mellitus will develop signs and symptoms of polyneuropathy, the number with diabetic neuropathy is huge. The symptoms of polyneuropathy are among the most common and debilitating complications of diabetes. In most patients with a diabetic polyneuropathy, sensory disturbances clearly predominate and progression of the polyneuropathy is slow (years). Sensory loss and autonomic dysfunction can lead to microtrauma and secondary foot ulcers, especially at pressure points (Figure 24.1).

Electrophysiological tests typically show features of an axonal neuropathy and provide no clues as to another diagnosis. It is debatable whether diabetic patients with a typical diabetic polyneuropathy according to the case history and neurological examination require electrophysiological investigations for diagnostic purposes. EMG will probably show a mild axonal neuropathy but provide no clue as to a causative diagnosis. Further laboratory examination including EMG is required to rule out other causes of the polyneuropathy in certain circumstances (Table 24.1).

If a patient with a polyneuropathy is not diagnosed with diabetes, a consensus report has suggested

Table 24.1. Indications for further laboratory examination including electromyography in patients with diabetes mellitus and neuropathy to rule out other causes of the polyneuropathy

- More rapidly progressive course
- Predominant motor neuropathy
- Asymmetry
- Severe pain early in the course of disease
- Clear autonomic disturbances
- Family history of polyneuropathy
- Any other doubt about a typical diabetic polyneuropathy

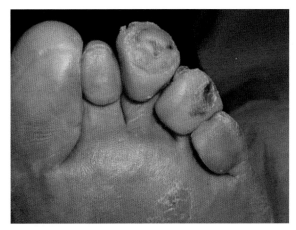

Figure 24.1. Secondary foot ulcers, especially at pressure points due to reduced or absent sensation causing neurogenic "diabetic foot."

that several screening laboratory tests may be considered (Level C evidence). Tests that provide the highest diagnostic yield were blood glucose level, serum vitamin B12 concentration, and serum protein immunofixation for M-protein. If there is no definite evidence of diabetes mellitus by routine testing of blood glucose, testing for impaired glucose tolerance may be considered in distal symmetric sensory polyneuropathy.

Polyneuropathy in patients with diabetes is often painful. The symptoms may require treatment with antiepileptic drugs – most evidence for a positive effect has been obtained with pregabalin, or amitriptyline, starting with a low dose, especially in elderly patients. Treatment of a painful neuropathy is difficult. When the suggested strategies fail, several drugs (such as other antiepileptic drugs) can be tried, but high-level evidence for a clear treatment effect often is absent. Several new drugs to treat painful neuropathy are under study currently.

Suggested reading

Bril V, England J, Franklin GM, et al. Evidence-based guideline: treatment of painful diabetic neuropathy: report of the American Academy of Neurology, the American Association of Neuromuscular and Electrodiagnostic Medicine, and the American Academy of Physical Medicine and Rehabilitation. *Neurology* 2011; **76**: 1758–1765.

Callaghan BC, Cheng HT, Stables CL, Smith AL, Feldman EL. Diabetic neuropathy: clinical manifestations and current treatments. *Lancet Neurol* 2012; **11**: 521–534.

England JD, Gronseth GS, Franklin G, et al. Practice Parameter: evaluation of distal symmetric polyneuropathy: role of laboratory and genetic testing (an evidence-based review). Report of the American Academy of Neurology, American Association of Neuromuscular and Electrodiagnostic Medicine, and American Academy of Physical Medicine and Rehabilitation. *Neurology* 2009; **72**: 185–192.

Zilliox L, Russell JW. Treatment of diabetic sensory polyneuropathy. *Curr Treat Options Neurol* 2011; **13**: 143–159.

Alcoholic neuropathy: a golf player with tingling feet who drank a bottle a day

Clinical history

A 66-year-old, retired bank manager was referred to our outpatient clinic because of slowly progressive tingling and numbness in his feet that had been present for two years. Walking became increasingly unpleasant as he constantly thought he had gravel in his shoes. He had problems keeping his balance after rising from a chair or from bed. He had no symptoms in his hands, and he did not notice weakness. He enjoyed playing golf several times a week, but had increasing difficulty finishing 18 holes. For years, he had been known to have a steatotic liver and hypertension. He did not smoke, but said that for many years he was used to drinking six glasses of beer or wine a day. He used antihypertensive drugs and vitamin B complex.

Examination

He was obese, had a highly colored face, and rather warm, red feet with a degree of hyperhydrosis. Neurological examination revealed a stocking-and-glove pattern diminished sensation of touch and pain in both hands and 15 cm distally from his knees. Vibration sense was lowered at the ankles and absent at the hallux. Position sense was normal. There was minor weakness of his anterior tibial and extensor hallucis muscles. Achilles tendon reflexes were reduced. The knee–heel test revealed minor ataxia. Romberg sign was weakly positive.

Ancillary investigations

Glucose level and kidney function were normal. Liver enzymes, especially gamma-GT, were elevated. He had no M-protein. Vitamin B1 and B6 levels were within normal limits (in particular, pyridoxine was not increased). Electrophysiological tests revealed an axonal, predominantly sensory polyneuropathy.

Diagnostic considerations and follow-up

The patient has a slowly progressive axonal polyneuropathy with a history and clinical signs compatible with excessive use of alcohol. Despite taking vitamin B complex, the patient developed the neuropathy. We strongly advised him to stop or to reduce his alcohol intake.

When we examined the patient a year later, he told us he had reduced his alcohol intake. There was no progression of the symptoms and signs of the polyneuropathy.

General remarks

Alcoholic polyneuropathy is characterized by the features of a predominantly distally located symmetric sensory neuropathy that can be painful with hyperesthesia and hyperpathia. Weakness may occur. Achilles tendon reflexes are reduced or absent, as can be expected in progressive axonal neuropathy. There are often associated features like thin and tender muscles, and autonomic features such as hyperhydrosis, especially in severe cases.

The etiology of alcoholic neuropathy has been debated for nearly a century. Initially, alcoholic neuropathy was considered to reflect a toxic neuropathy. In later years, vitamin B1 (thiamine) deficiency was thought to be the most likely explanation, as many alcoholics are malnourished and neuropathy in alcoholics shares many identical clinical, electrophysiological, and histopathological features with beriberi. It was hypothesized that alcohol affects thiamine utilization rather than causes thiamine deficiency. Thiamine treatment does not, however, with continued drinking reverse alcoholic neuropathy. Furthermore, ethanol neurotoxicity in the brain has been firmly established. New evidence from experimental studies suggests a similar toxic effect of ethanol on the peripheral nervous system.

The mechanism underlying alcoholic neuropathy is not well understood. Several explanations have been proposed, including activation of spinal cord microglia after chronic alcohol consumption, oxidative stress leading to free radical damage to nerves, activation of mGlu5 receptors in the spinal cord, and activation of the sympathoadrenal and hypothalamus–pituitary–adrenal (HPA) axis. In addition, pure thiamine deficiency neuropathy develops as a more acutely progressive motor-dominant neuropathy. It is not known why some people develop signs and symptoms of a polyneuropathy relatively rapidly. Genetic susceptibility to the development of alcoholic neuropathy cannot be excluded; other metabolic factors (metabolic syndrome) may play an additional role.

There is no exact data on the level of alcohol consumption required before the symptoms of an alcoholic neuropathy become manifest. Development of the disorder is correlated with the total amount of alcohol consumed throughout life and the duration of alcohol consumption. Patients taking >100 g of alcohol (about 5–7 glasses) per day over a period of several years, especially those who skip proper meals, are at risk. In conclusion, the cause of alcoholic neuropathy is most probably multifactorial with an important role for vitamin B1 deficiency, but the toxic effect of alcohol may be more important. Metabolic factors can play a role as do impurities such as lead in wine.

Laboratory investigation should check for anemia, liver enzyme changes, vitamin B1 level, and erythrocyte transketolase activity. Electrophysiological tests typically reveal features of an axonal length-dependent neuropathy with mild to moderate reduction of compound muscle action potentials and moderate slowing of motor nerve conduction, compatible with secondary demyelination as a consequence of axonal degeneration. Sensory nerve action potentials are severely reduced.

Treatment consists of:

- Vitamin B1 supplementation (1–3 times per day, 50 mg thiamine orally; in severe cases start with 100 mg thiamine subcutaneously or intramuscularly) and vitamin B complex

- Cessation of drinking alcohol or at least reducing the amount of alcohol consumption
- Switching to a proper diet when indicated
- Symptomatic treatment of pain and dysesthesias with amitriptyline, gabapentin, or pregabalin

Symptoms and signs may remain stable or partially disappear over a period of months. It should be kept in mind that, as in most axonal neuropathies, the first aim must be to halt progression. If the neuropathy clearly worsens over time, continuous alcohol over-consumption, metabolic factors like diabetes, but also vitamin B6 (pyridoxine) intoxication should be considered.

Suggested reading

Ang CD, Alviar MJM, Dans AL, et al. Vitamin B for treating peripheral neuropathy. *Cochrane Database Syst Rev* 2008; **3**: CD004573.

Koike H, Sobue G. Alcoholic neuropathy. *Curr Opin Neurol* 2006; **19**: 481–486.

Manji H. Toxic neuropathy. *Curr Opin Neurol* 2011; **24**: 484–490.

Mellion M, Gilchrist JM, de la Monte S. Alcohol-related peripheral neuropathy: nutritional, toxic, or both. *Muscle Nerve* 2011; **43**: 309–316.

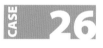

Human immunodeficiency virus neuropathy: a man with pain in the lower legs that hampered proper walking

Clinical history

A 48-year-old man complained of a dull feeling and tingling sensations in both feet, that over a period of months crept upward toward the knees. Gradually the character of these sensations converted to pain, especially when touching the skin, and wearing socks and shoes. Human immune deficiency (HIV) infection had been diagnosed three years previously. Since then, he had been treated with antiretroviral therapy.

Examination

The neurological examination of the cranial nerves and arms was normal. Below the knees he had impaired pain, touch, vibration, and position senses. No weakness was found. The Achilles tendon reflexes were absent. He had mild rombergism and a broad-based walking pattern. The knee–heel test, however, was normal.

Ancillary investigations

He was HIV-positive with a CD4 count of 0.6 (normal). EMG revealed a sensory axonal neuropathy with normal concentric needle analysis and motor nerve conduction velocities.

Diagnostic considerations and follow-up

HIV-associated distal symmetric polyneuropathy (DSP) was diagnosed. No other cause was found.

Initially, he was treated with amitriptyline without effect. Following treatment with lamotrigine, the pain almost disappeared. The findings were largely unchanged when he was examined four years later. At that time, he had complaints suggesting a carpal tunnel syndrome. The pain in the legs persisted at low intensity, especially when being touched.

General remarks

Neuromuscular disorders are common in HIV (Table 26.1). HIV-associated DSP occurs in 40%–50% of patients. Several other neuropathies can occur, depending on the stage of infection. In the early course of the disease, these include both GBS and CIDP, especially at the time of seroconversion. In contrast to patients with idiopathic forms of GBS and CIDP, HIV patients with these neuropathies have high CSF cell counts ($>50 \times 10^6$/L). As a consequence, marked pleocytosis in patients with otherwise probable idiopathic GBS or CIDP justifies diagnostic tests for HIV.

Multifocal neuropathies due to necrotizing vasculitis may occur at a later stage of HIV infection. Opportunistic infections such as with cytomegalovirus (CMV) also occur later. Polyradiculoneuropathy with increased CSF count can be extremely painful.

DSP remains a major cause of morbidity in HIV-infected patients, antiretroviral drug toxicity adding to its development. Newer anti-HIV drugs are less harmful and the independent risk of protease inhibitors seems to be low. The potential side effects of these drugs must, however, be balanced against their important role in antiretroviral therapeutic regimens. The pathogenesis of HIV-associated DSP is not completely understood.

Table 26.1. Neuromuscular disorders in human immunodeficiency virus infection

Disorder	Characteristic features	Diagnostic tests	Treatment
DSP	Numbness, pain, paresthesias Stocking-and-glove distribution Sensory >> motor Vibration sense (near) normal Motor features occur late (feet) Ankle reflexes hypoactive Slow progression	EMG: axonal neuropathy Exclude other causes CSF analysis and sural nerve biopsy not indicated	Management of neuropathic pain: anticonvulsants; antidepressants; nonspecific analgesics: all disappointing Topical (capsaicin); smoking cannabis
GBS and CIDP	Clinically indistinguishable from GBS and CIDP in non-HIV Occur at time of seroconversion	CSF: mild pleocytosis; protein elevated If serum CD4 <200: exclude infection/malignancy	IVIg
Entrapment mononeuropathies	HIV patients at risk	Similar to non-HIV patients	Symptomatic
Facial palsy	Idiopathic (Bell's palsy) at any stage: as in non-HIV patients	CSF (exclude other etiologies)	If no cause, five days course of steroids
	Ramsay Hunt syndrome: VZV	CSF	Acyclovir; effect of steroids uncertain
Mononeuropathy multiplex	Multifocal deficit < nerve infarction Associated with AIDS and CMV	EMG CMV diagnosis (CSF: PCR)	Antiviral: ganiclovir, foscarnet, cidofovir
Progressive radiculopathy	CMV infection of cauda equina, and lumbosacral nerve root Rapid progression	MRI with gadolineum CMV diagnosis (CSF: PCR) Exclude neurosyphilis, lymphoma, EBV	Antiviral: ganiclovir, foscarnet, cidofovir
HIV-associated polymyositis	Limb girdle weakness, myalgia	CK elevation, myopathic EMG Myopathic muscle biopsy	Corticosteroids and other immunosuppressants Immunomodulation
Toxic myopathy associated with antiretroviral therapy	Weakness, exercise intolerance	Ragged red fibers in muscle biopsy (mitochondrial dysfunction)	Improvement after withdrawal of causative drug

Adapted from Robinson-Papp J, Simpson DM. Neuromuscular diseases associated with HIV-1 infection. *Muscle Nerve* 2009; **40**: 1043–1053. EBV, Epstein–Barr virus; PCR, polymerase chain reaction; VZV, *Varicella zoster* virus.

A role for HIV-infected macrophages that secrete neurotoxic mediators in DRG has been demonstrated. In addition, pathological and experimental evidence suggests that mitochondrial dysfunction in distal axons contributes to the development of HIV-associated sensory neuropathy. In patients who have died from HIV-associated complications, distal sensory nerve segments showed increased levels of common deletions of mitochondrial DNA compared with DRG. Healthy controls showed no deletions of mitochondrial DNA. Treatment with antiretroviral drugs may play a causative role.

DSP, which is usually painful, occurs in 40%–50% of HIV patients. As it is so common in HIV patients and as it has no specific features, other causes of sensory neuropathy such as diabetes, alcohol intoxication, hypothyroidism, and vitamin B12 deficiency must be excluded. Even with successful antiretroviral therapy, DSP remains prevalent, causing substantial disability and reduced quality of life. Lamotrigine and local capsaicine treatment appear effective, at least in a proportion of patients.

Suggested reading

Ellis RJ, Marquie-Beck J, Delaney P, et al. Human immunodeficiency virus protease inhibitors and risk for peripheral neuropathy. *Ann Neurol* 2008; **64**: 566–572.

Ellis RJ, Rosario D, Clifford DB, et al. Continued high prevalence and adverse clinical impact of human immunodeficiency virus-associated sensory neuropathy in the era of combination antiretroviral therapy. *Arch Neurol* 2010; **67**: 552–558.

Gonzalez-Duarte A, Robinson-Papp J, Simpson DM. Diagnosis and management of HIV-associated neuropathy. *Neurol Clin* 2008; **26**: 821–832.

Lehmann HC, Chen W, Borzan J, Mankowski JL, Hoke A. Mitochondrial dysfunction in distal axons contributes to human immunodefiency virus sensory neuropathy. *Ann Neurol* 2011; **69**: 100–110.

Robinson-Papp J, Simpson DM. Neuromuscular diseases associated with HIV-infection. *Muscle Nerve* 2009; **40**: 1043–1053.

CASE 27 Lyme radiculoneuritis: a 56-year-old man with abdominal pain

Clinical history

In December, the patient experienced abdominal pains and constipation. The following April, while on vacation in France, his complaints worsened and feces had to be removed manually. Coloscopy did not reveal any abnormality and the gastroenterologist did not find an explanation for his discomfort. He had been a heavy drinker until type 2 diabetes mellitus was diagnosed. In June, when he developed facial asymmetry and acute pain in his lower legs, we were consulted in the Accident and Emergency Department. He mentioned malaise and areas of decreased sensation on his back. He did not recall a tick bite or erythema migrans (EM).

Examination

We noted incomplete peripheral facial nerve palsy on the right side of his face, hypesthesia in the left C6 dermatome with absent triceps tendon reflex on the same side, and decreased sensation in the T4–T10 area with absent abdominal skin reflexes. The most striking feature was bilateral protrusion of his abdominal wall (Figure 27.1), more pronounced on the left side. He could not rise from the supine position without using his hands.

Ancillary investigations

The MRI of his spine was normal. A CT scan revealed thin abdominal wall muscles, but no other abnormalities (Figure 27.2). EMG showed denervation activity without reinnervation potentials in muscles innervated by T2–L4 spinal roots. Denervation was absent in bulbar and cervical regions. CSF analysis showed mononuclear pleocytosis of 80×10^6/L (<4/L) cells with a protein level of 1.42 g/L (<0.4). The high IgG-index of 0.77 and multiple oligoclonal bands suggested intrathecal synthesis of immunoglobulins.

Using ELISA and immunoblots, serum IgG and IgM antibodies against *Borrelia burgdorferi* were demonstrated. CSF ELISA also showed IgG and IgM antibodies.

A B

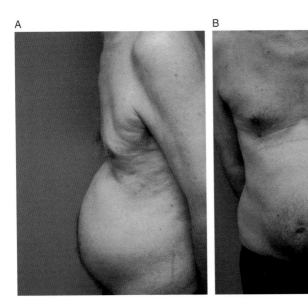

Figure 27.1. (A, B) Bilateral, asymmetric protrusion of abdominal wall.

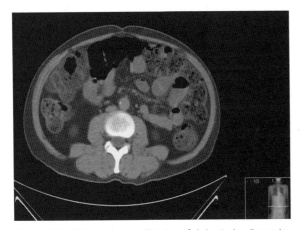

Figure 27.2. CT scan showing thinning of abdominal wall muscles resulting from chronic denervation.

Diagnostic considerations

Serology for other infectious agents proved negative and autoimmune diseases were excluded by appropriate tests. We diagnosed abdominal pseudohernia with constipation and abdominal pains due to abdominal wall muscle weakness caused by spinal lymphocytic meningoradiculitis. Tick-borne lymphocytic meningoradiculitis, Bannwarth syndrome, is a European manifestation of Lyme neuroborreliosis. The onset was probably six months prior to diagnosis and symptoms increased gradually. The patient did not recall EM. He received a four-week course of intravenous ceftriaxone. After five months, abdominal pains had

disappeared, but muscle weakness remained. Constipation was avoided by using laxatives.

General remarks

Tick-borne meningitis, cranial neuritis, and lymphocytic meningoradiculitis are usually caused by infection with the spirochaete *B. burgdorferi*. Ticks, however, can be infected with other microorganisms that may cause neurological or systemic disease. Coinfection of ticks with *Babesia microti*, *Anaplasma phagocyrophilum*, *Ehrlichia*, and tick-borne encephalitis virus, in addition to the *B. burgdorferi* species, has been reported.

Ticks have a four-stage life cycle–egg, larva, nymph, and adult–feeding only once during every stage. In the wild, ticks live on birds, rodents, and deer. Most infections in humans are caused by bites of small nymphs that escape detection. Ixodic ticks, that can transmit *B. burgdorferi* to humans, live in the mild climate zones of eastern and western parts of North America, Eurasia, and the Middle East. The percentage of ticks that are infected with *B. burgdorferi* varies between regions and countries.

Borrelia genospecies, time of exposure, and the local immune response of the host determine whether a bite from an infected tick causes infection. Lyme neuroborreliosis in North America is caused by *B. burgdorferi sensu stricto*. In Europe, at least five species of Lyme *Borrelia* have been implicated. Genetic variations between *Borrelia* genospecies explain the variety

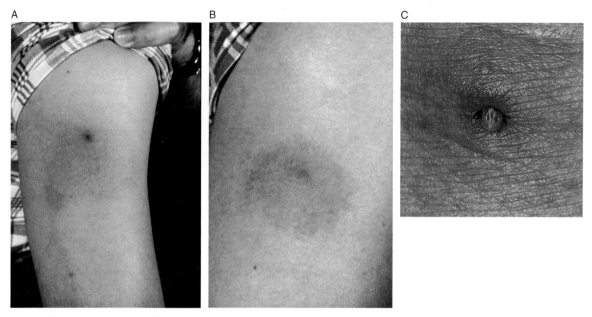

Figure 27.3. Erythema migrans (EM) is an area of expanding erythema with a diameter of at least 5 cm (A). EM is pathognomonic for Lyme disease. It can be raised a little and somewhat bluish. During a few days to weeks, EM will expand (B). Sometimes a tick can be observed *in situ* (C).

of clinical symptoms of infection between North American and European patients. In Europe, most infected patients develop EM around the site of the bite (Figure 27.3). In North America, EM and lymphocytic meningoradiculitis appear less frequently.

Annual incidence rates of all manifestations in selected areas in Europe range between 69 and 315 per 100 000. In one German study, 89% had EM; 5% had arthritis, and less than 1% carditis. Only 3% had early Lyme neuroborreliosis, suggesting an incidence of around three per 100 000.

Most cases of EM have been reported from late May until late September. Neurological and other signs of disseminated disease can occur throughout the year. Antecedent EM is not usually reported in Lyme neuroborreliosis. Few patients recall a tick bite. Cardiac conduction abnormalities can also be a feature of acute Lyme disease (see Table 38.1).

Neurological manifestations are caused by infection and mild to moderate inflammation of the subarachnoid space and perineural tissue. As Lyme neuroborreliosis usually develops over a period of weeks, most patients have a diagnostic delay. Syndromes include spinal and cranial meningoradiculitis, acute usually axonal poly- or mononeuritis, plexus neuritis, and chronic meningitis, especially in children. Cranial nerves, most frequently the facial nerve, can be implicated. Radicular pain can be

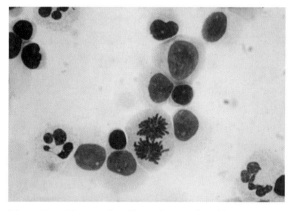

Figure 27.4. Mitotic cell and large plasma cells in CSF (May–Grünwald Giemsa staining).

excruciating, but may be absent. Rare manifestations of neuroborreliosis include myelitis and localized myositis, and extremely rarely in the case of late Lyme neuroborreliosis, cerebral vasculitis. Symmetric chronic neuropathy is not a manifestation of Lyme disease.

Diagnosis of Lyme neuroborreliosis is based on four pillars: history, neurological examination, analysis of CSF including the IgG-index and presence of oligoclonal banding pattern, and antibody studies of serum and CSF. The CSF may contain immature cells and large plasma cells, suggesting a hematological malignancy (Figure 27.4). For serological diagnosis, a two-step approach is advocated, the first step being an ELISA. If positive, an IgG and IgM immunoblot assay should confirm the diagnosis. Tests can be negative in early disease and remain positive following treatment. Background seropositivity ranges between 4% in endemic areas and 50% in asymptomatic Austrian hunters. Many of them have never been ill. As neurological manifestations present weeks to months after initial infection, serological tests are usually positive. A high antibody index in CSF compared with serum is the mainstay of serological diagnosis of Lyme neuroborreliosis.

Standard therapy for neuroborreliosis consists of a two- to four-week course of intravenous ceftriaxone or penicillin. Recovery is usually prompt, but axonal damage can lead to persisting signs. Some patients without evidence of persisting infection may develop a post-Lyme disease syndrome that can be characterized by persisting fatigue, musculoskeletal pain, difficulties with concentration and memory,

and sleep problems. Re-treatment with antibiotics does not have a favorable effect in these patients.

Suggested reading

Lantos PM, Charini WA, Medoff G, et al. Final report of the Lyme disease review panel of the infectious disease society of America. *Clin Infect Dis* 2010; **51**: 1–5.

Mygland A, Ljøstad U, Fingerle V, et al. EFNS guidelines on the diagnosis and management of European Lyme neuroborreliosis. *Eur J Neurol* 2010; **17**: 8–16.

Oschmann P, Dorndorf W, Hornig C, et al. Stages of neuroborreliosis. *J Neurol* 1998; **245**: 262–272.

Pachner AR, Steiner I. Lyme neuroborreliosis: infection, immunity, and inflammation. *Lancet Neurol* 2007; **6**: 544–552.

Stanek G, Wormser GP, Gray J, Strle F. Lyme borreliosis. *Lancet* 2012; **379**: 461–473.

www.cdc.gov/lyme/

CASE 28 — Lepromatous neuropathy: a girl with progressive weakness of one hand

Clinical history

A 14-year-old girl (born in Brazil, moved to Europe at a young age) presented with weakness and a dull feeling in her right hand. The symptoms had been progressive over a period of one year. Initially, she had diminished sensation in her right index finger. This gradually progressed to affect the whole of her right hand, which eventually became numb. She is right-handed and could no longer write. Otherwise her history was unremarkable.

Examination

She had a claw hand with atrophy of the intrinsic muscles of the right hand (Figure 28.1). There was a paresis (MRC grade 2–4) of all hand muscles innervated by the median, ulnar, and radial nerves. She had sensory disturbances of all modalities with the exception of the position sense. The biceps, brachioradial, and triceps reflexes were diminished in the right arm. On palpation, the ulnar, median, and radial nerves on the right side appeared to be enlarged. We noticed some changes in

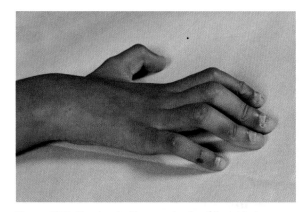

Figure 28.1. Claw hand with some atrophy of the intrinsic muscles. Damage to the tip of the index finger and nail beds is due to wounds following loss of sensation.

the color of the distal part of her right arm, compatible with depigmentation. There were no abnormalities of the left arm and the legs. Because leprosy was considered, she consulted a dermatologist.

Ancillary investigations

When we first investigated the patient, routine blood examination and an MRI of the cervical spine and brachial plexus had already been performed by the referring neurologist. None of the tests revealed abnormalities. Ultrasound imaging demonstrated enlarged nerves in the arms. The skin biopsy of the depigmented lesion showed a perivascular and periadnexal infiltrate and granuloma formation, which was compatible with leprosy (Figure 28.2).

Diagnostic considerations

The initial differential diagnosis included a middle or lower brachial plexus lesion, a cervical syrinx, HNPP, MADSAM neuropathy, and leprosy. Leprosy was suggested by the combination of the enlarged nerves with hypopigmented skin lesions and diffuse motor and sensory disturbances of one hand.

Follow-up

Once the patient had been diagnosed with leprosy of the bordeline-tuberculoid type, treatment with dapsone, rifampicine, clofazamine, and prednisolone was started. After several months of treatment, while sensory disturbances had partially disappeared, she burned her hand when using a hairdryer. The muscles of her right hand were trained by a hand physical therapist and it appeared that there was some increase in muscle function over a period of one year.

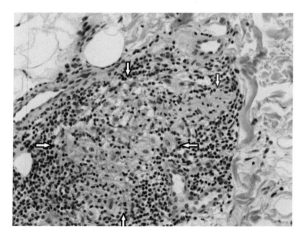

Figure 28.2. Skin biopsy of depigmented lesion: white arrows indicate the perivascular and periadnexal infiltrate and granuloma formation; red arrow identifies a dermal nerve.

General remarks

Every year, about 200 000 new leprosy cases are diagnosed worldwide. In Europe and North America, the incidence is low. When recording the case history, information about migration must be included, as more than 80% of all registered leprosy cases are from India, Brazil, Burma, Indonesia, Madagascar, and Nepal.

Leprosy is caused by a chronic granulomatous immune response to infection of the skin and nerves with *Mycobacterium leprae*, which resides in macrophages and Schwann cells. Nerve damage, affecting mainly the ulnar, median, and posterior tibial nerves, results in nerve enlargement. As the replication time of *M. leprae* is slow, the incubation period can range from a few years to over 30 years (mean 2–7 years). *M. leprae* can penetrate nerves presumably by binding to laminin, and very often causes signs of neuropathy. As the optimal replication temperature of *M. leprae* is low, it is probable that it will preferentially affect the more superficial parts of nerves. Subsequently, enlarged nerves are more vulnerable to compression. In combination with inflammation and the formation of granulomata, this could easily produce symptoms and signs of mononeuropathy, multiple mononeuropathy (most frequent), or polyneuropathy. The peripheral nerves that are usually affected are – in order – the posterior tibial nerve, ulnar, median, and peroneal nerve.

Leprosy is a clinical diagnosis requiring the presence of at least one of the following: a hypopigmented or erythromatous skin lesion with a local hypesthesic area through involvement of dermal nerves, involvement of peripheral nerves (enlarged nerves on clinical examination and high-resolution sonography), or the identification of *M. leprae* in a biopsy from a depigmented lesion or sural nerve. The primary goal of leprosy treatment with dapsone, rifampicin, minocycline, and other drugs is to stop the active infection with *M. leprae* in order to avoid progressive inflammation and the formation of granulomata. Rehabilitation and physical therapy may help to improve muscle weakness. Education is important in order to prevent further damage due to (burn) wounds.

Suggested reading

Jacobson RR, Krahenbuhl JL. Leprosy. *Lancet* 1999; **353**: 655–660.

Jain S, Visser LH, Praveen TLN, et al. High-resolution sonography: a new technique to detect nerve damage in leprosy. *PLoS Negl Trop Dis* 2009; **3**: e498.

WHO Expert Committee on Leprosy. *World Health Organ Tech Rep Ser* 1998; **874**: 1–43.

Toxic iatrogenic neuropathy: a man with a blue face and a polyneuropathy following myocardial infarction

Clinical history

A 76-year-old man complained about progressive dull feelings and weakness of the distal lower limbs that gradually progressed over a couple of months to the proximal legs and the hands. He was known to have suffered a myocardial infarction and cardiac arrhythmia three years previously. Since then, he had been treated with amiodarone. He had no visual complaints and was otherwise healthy.

Examination

The patient had problems rising from a chair and walking was difficult. We found diffuse weakness of muscles in both arms and legs, more pronounced distally (MRC grade 4) than proximally. He had minor distal stocking-and-glove sensory disturbances and areflexia. Tremor and gait ataxia were absent. Furthermore, he had a somewhat blue-grayish discoloration of his face that suggested a relationship with amiodarone.

Ancillary investigations

Routine blood investigation was normal. No M-protein was found. EMG showed signs of a demyelinating polyneuropathy. Because of this finding, a diagnosis of CIDP was considered (Case 16). CSF revealed a slightly elevated protein (0.7 g/L) without pleocytosis. A sural nerve biopsy indicated signs of demyelination with membrane-bound osmophilic inclusions, compatible with an amiodarone-related neuropathy.

Follow-up

Amiodarone was stopped. The neuropathy gradually improved over the course of about one year. When he was seen four years later, he was in good health and symptoms and signs of neuropathy were almost absent. The blue-grayish discoloration of his face had virtually disappeared.

General remarks

Toxic iatrogenic neuropathies can be axonal and demyelinating (Table 29.1). Neuropathies can be caused by a variety of drugs and toxic substances (Table 29.2). It is important to consider toxic

Table 29.1. Examples of toxic neuropathies

Axonal neuropathy

Acrylamide, alcohol, arsenic, bortezomib, colchicine, dapsone, dioxin, disulfiram, ethambutol, IFN-alpha, isoniazid, lead, lithium, metronidazole, nitrofurantoin, organophosphates, phenytoin, platinum analogs, pyridoxine, statins, taxol, vinca alkaloids

Demyelinating neuropathy

Amiodarone, chloroquine, tacrolimus, perhexiline, procainamide, zelmidine

Table 29.2. Cytostatic drugs that may cause polyneuropathy

Agent	Symptoms and signs	Reversible after discontinuation
Bortezomib	Sensory, painful	Gradually
Paclitaxel (Taxol)	Paresthesias, dysesthesias (weakness), ataxia	Partially
Vincristine	Sensorimotor and autonomic	Yes
Cisplatin	Sensory axonopathy, ataxia (neuronopathy), L'hermitte sign	May worsen after discontinuation

The relationship between the occurrence of neuropathy and the use of cytostatic drugs is usually dose-related.

If axonal or neuronal degeneration has occurred, permanent symptoms and signs remain.

etiologies in the differential diagnosis of neuropathies, because they are among the treatable forms of peripheral nerve dysfunction. When examining and evaluating a patient with a polyneuropathy, one of the important questions to ask is about the use of cytostatics or other drugs. A large number of drugs can cause neuropathy, some of which are not used very frequently. Especially when the full side-effect profile is not very well known, one should check whether a drug could be associated with the development of polyneuropathy. It is remarkable that chronic use of high dosage vitamin B6 (pyridoxine) can induce a mainly sensory and ataxic neuropathy. The precise mechanism is not well understood.

Toxic neuropathies most frequently induce pure sensory or sensorimotor symptoms. Pain can be a prominent feature. Most toxic neuropathies are

A
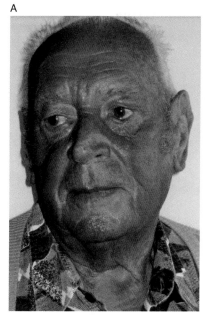

B
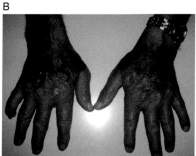

Figure 29.1. Blue discoloration of the skin of the face and hands due to amiodarone. Exposure to sunlight causes more bluish discoloration. (From Stähli BE, Schwab S. Amiodarone-induced skin hyperpigmentation *QJM* 2011; **104**: 723–724, with permission.)

axonal or predominantly axonal. Some can, however, be (predominantly) demyelinating and may mimic CIDP. Amiodarone neuropathy is one of these. The overt proximal weakness that can also occur in amiodarone neuropathy may resemble CIDP. A blue discoloration of the skin – especially after sun exposure – is a well-known side effect of amiodarone (Figure 29.1). It has been explained by the accumulation of lipofuscine, or deposits of electron-dense granules and can disappear after discontinuation of amiodarone.

Optic neuropathy occurs in 1%–2% of patients who are treated with amiodarone. Peripheral neuropathy is less prevalent. As with most toxic neuropathies, it has been shown that the chance of developing an amiodarone-related neuropathy is dependent on the dose and duration of treatment.

Stopping amiodarone can result in virtual disappearance of the neuropathy. When informing a patient, one should bear in mind that progression of symptoms and signs of neuropathy may continue for three to six months after cessation of the causative agent. This is the so-called coasting effect.

Suggested reading

Orr CF, Ahslkog JE. Frequency, characteristics, and risk factors for amiodarone neurotoxicity. *Arch Neurol* 2009; **66**: 865–869.

Vassallo P, Trohman RG. Prescribing amiodarone: an evidence-based review of clinical indications. *JAMA* 2007; **298**: 1312–1322.

Windebank AJ, Grisold W. Chemotherapy-induced neuropathy. *J Periph Nerv Syst* 2008; **13**: 27–46.

Idiopathic neuralgic amyotrophy: a stand fitter with frequent shoulder dislocations following extreme shoulder pain

Clinical history

A 19-year-old stand fitter experienced acute, stinging pain in the upper region of the left arm that reached a maximum in one day and prevented him from sleeping for one week. The pain did not radiate into the arm or toward the neck. It increased when he lifted his left arm. Analgesics and an injection by his GP, who suggested bursitis, had no effect. He could not work for five weeks. During this period, the pain gradually subsided only to increase when he held the steering wheel of his car. He did not notice weakness or disturbed sensation. The family history was negative.

Examination

On examination in a regional hospital, he was found to have atrophy of the left rhomboid, supraspinatus, and infraspinatus muscles (Figure 30.1), and weakness, MRC grade 4, of the supraspinatus and infraspinatus muscles. Sensation and reflexes were normal.

Ancillary investigations

Laboratory analysis of the blood did not support a diagnosis of diabetes or autoimmune disease. Serum antibodies to *Borrelia burgdorferi* were negative. He had no CSF pleocytosis. An MRI scan of the brachial plexus was also normal. At referral after eight months, EMG was abnormal with fibrillation potentials and positive sharp waves, but no fasciculation in the

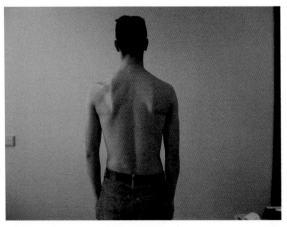

Figure 30.1. Atrophy of left rhomboid, supraspinatus, and infraspinatus muscles as residual features of a patient with idiopathic neuralgic amyotrophy.

supraspinatus and infraspinatus muscles. Needle EMG of the infraspinatus, deltoid, and biceps brachii muscles showed neurogenic MUPs. The left antebrachial cutaneous nerve SNAP (part of the musculocutaneous nerve, C6) was decreased.

Diagnostic considerations

The patient had overt signs of involvement of the C5 and C6 nerve roots, or alternatively the suprascapular, axillary, and musculocutaneous nerves (See Introduction, Table 13). The rhomboid muscle is innervated by the dorsal scapular nerve (C5). Involvement of multiple nerves and/or nerve roots strongly suggests plexus neuropathy. Acute painful onset with subsequent weakness to follow and no cause identified suggests a diagnosis of idiopathic neuralgic amyotrophy (INA), brachial plexus neuritis of the upper part of the brachial plexus.

Follow-up

He could gradually return to work, but in subsequent months to years he experienced frequent painless dislocations of the left humerus. This could occur twice a week, or only once in six months. Risk factors were unexpected movements, working with his arms raised above his head, and forcefully pulling objects with his arms either above his head or while reaching downward. He could easily reposition the humerus. After long working hours he experienced dull musculoskeletal pain in the left shoulder region. Because of these habitual dislocations, he could no longer play football.

Neurological examination after nine years showed atrophy of the infraspinatus and rhomboid muscles and mild weakness, MRC grade 4–5, of the infraspinatus muscle.

General remarks

INA is, by definition, an acute, very painful upper brachial plexopathy, usually with winged scapula and no cause identified. The reported incidence is 2–3/100 000 per year. The male: female ratio is about 2:1. Most patients experience a single period of INA, but the chance of recurrence varies between 5% and 26%.

Neuralgic amyotrophy, also known as Parsonage–Turner syndrome, can occur as an AD hereditary trait, hereditary neuralgic amyotrophy (HNA). About half of the families show mutations in the septin-9 (SEPT9) gene. HNA is thought to be 10 times less common than INA. Patients with HNA have earlier onset (28 versus 41 years), more attacks, and more frequent involvement of nerves outside the brachial plexus (56% versus 17%) than patients with INA. Weakness may also be more severe and functional outcome worse. On a single patient level, no clinical or diagnostic test, mutation analysis excepted, can discriminate between INA and HNA. After a first attack of INA in sporadic patients, mutation analysis of the SEPT9 gene is not advised as a negative test does not rule out heredity.

INA is characterized by initially severe, continuous stabbing or shooting pain – usually worse at night – for an average of four weeks (range: 1–60 days). A minority of patients have pain with stuttering onset that may switch on and off before worsening. Only a small minority of patients reports no pain.

Sensory involvement – hypesthetic skin areas usually with a patchy distribution with loss not according to dermatomes – occurs in 80% of patients, but is less prominent compared to the paresis that follows after the pain subsides. INA is a patchy disorder and may affect any nerve in the brachial plexus. Damage in the upper and middle trunk with involvement of the long thoracic and/or suprascapular nerves appears most frequently. Motor abnormalities in INA form a spectrum. At one extreme, unilateral neuropathy of the interosseus anterior nerve (a median nerve branch) or the posterior interosseus nerve (a radial nerve branch) can be affected. At the other end of the spectrum, one finds bilateral brachial plexus neuropathy with severe arm weakness and orthopnea due to diaphragm weakness resulting from phrenic nerve paralysis. Lumbosacral plexus neuropathy and recurrent laryngeal nerve involvement with hoarseness form part of the spectrum. Horner's sign is extremely rare. Predominant lower trunk involvement causes distal neuralgic amyotrophy with sympathetic nerve dysfunction leading to dysesthesia and vasomotor changes of the affected forearm and hand.

An autoimmune origin of INA has been suggested but all tests aimed at identifying a cause have proven negative. Mild CSF pleocytosis and patchy hyperintense T2 lesions on brachial plexus MRI scans may occur in the acute phase. Appropriate tests must be applied to exclude other causes of brachial plexus neuropathy, which include structural lesions of the lung, especially Pancoast tumor, cervical spine metastasis, brachial plexus nerve tumors, neurosarcoidosis, autoimmune vasculitis, and inflammatory radiculitis as in Lyme disease and HIV patients. Herpes zoster rash may be followed after a period ranging from one day to four months by focal motor weakness mimicking the pattern of INA. Lumbosacral plexopathy is a common complication of type 1 and type 2 diabetes mellitus and is called diabetic radiculoplexoneuropathy, Bruns–Garland syndrome. Interestingly, brachial plexopathy is not associated with diabetes.

Motor nerve conduction studies can be indicated to differentiate INA from HNPP, MMN, and variants of CIDP. Pain is usually absent in these conditions. Another indication for EMG is to detect which peripheral nerves are affected.

There is no evidence from systematic studies that supports efficacy of corticosteroids, but as contraindications are absent, these can be tried shortly after onset of pain. Unfortunately, diagnostic delay is usually much longer. Recovery may continue for up to two years after the attack, but many patients have persisting disability and pain. At follow-up, about a quarter of the patients are found to suffer from neuropathic pain. In particular, the glenohumeral joint is vulnerable to residual symptoms. Dysfunction includes paresis of the rotator cuff muscles with decreased glenohumeral excursions, frozen shoulder, and glenohumeral subluxation. The rotator cuff is formed by the supraspinatus, infraspinatus, teres minor, and subscapularis muscles (see Introduction, Table 13). Residual complaints after distal INA may include wrist or finger contractures.

Suggested reading

Steiner I, Kennedy PGE, Pachner A. The neurotropic herpes viruses: herpes simplex and varicella zoster. *Lancet Neurol* 2007; **6**: 1015–1028.

Van Alfen N. Clinical and pathophysiological concepts of neuralgic amyotrophy. *Nat Rev Neurol* 2011; 7: 315–322.

Van Alfen N, Van Engelen BGM. The clinical spectrum of neuralgic amyotrophy in 246 cases. *Brain* 2006; **129**: 438–450.

Small nerve fiber neuropathy: a marathon runner who could no longer run because of painful feet

Clinical history

A 48-year-old man had complained about painful feet for several months. This pain was present constantly, but increased when his soles were touched and when walking. He did not report weakness or sensory disturbances, nor discoloration of his feet or swelling of his joints. Otherwise he was healthy.

To be more specific, he was not known to have diabetes mellitus or any other chronic disorder, such as sarcoidosis, that could cause painful neuropathy (Table 31.1). Signs that could suggest malignancy were absent. He did not use medication, did not smoke, and drank only very limited amounts of alcohol. He was a marathon runner, but could no longer train or walk properly because of very painful feet. He did not have symptoms of autonomic neuropathy. There was no family history of neurological disorders.

Examination

Neurological examination was normal. On inspection, his feet looked normal, no discolorations of the skin or abnormal joints or tendons were observed, and he did not show clinical signs of autonomic failure. There were no sensory disturbances, except for the fact that touching the soles of his feet was extremely painful. In particular, the tendon reflexes were normal. He had no orthostatic hypotension.

Ancillary investigations

Routine serological examination revealed no abnormalities; in particular, fasting glucose and ESR were normal, and there were no liver or kidney function disturbances. There was no evidence of sarcoidosis. He had no M-protein. Extensive EMG examination was normal. Detailed quantitative sensory testing was not performed.

His principal complaint was extreme, distal pain suggestive of polyneuropathy. Definite evidence of neuropathy was absent. As no other explanation for painful feet, such as erythromelalgia or arthritis, was found, a diagnosis of idiopathic small nerve fiber was considered. Therefore, a skin biopsy was taken (Figure 31.1). A reduced number of intraepidermal nerve fibers (small nerve fibers) was observed compatible with a diagnosis of small fiber neuropathy (Figure 31.2).

Diagnostic considerations and follow-up

We could not identify a cause of the small fiber neuropathy (SFN). He was treated with several drugs for painful neuropathy with limited success.

General remarks

SFN often results in symptoms of burning pain, shooting pain, allodynia, and hyperesthesia. Diagnosis of SFN is

Table 31.1. Causes of small nerve fiber, painful sensory neuropathy

Metabolic	Diabetes mellitus
Toxic	Alcoholism, drugs (statins, nitrofurantoin)
Inflammatory	Paraneoplastic: sarcoidosis, Sjögren syndrome
Infectious	HIV
Hematological	cryoglobulinemia, primary amyloidosis
Genetic	Fabry disease SCN9A (sodium channel) gene-related (prominent dyasautonomia) HSAN
Idiopathic (I-SFN)	No cause yet identified

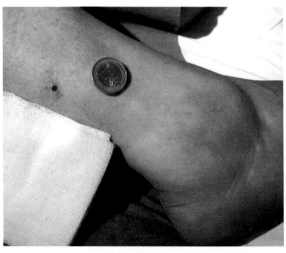

Figure 31.1. Location on outer ankle where skin biopsies can be taken. Note the small size of the biopsy compared with the one Euro coin.

A

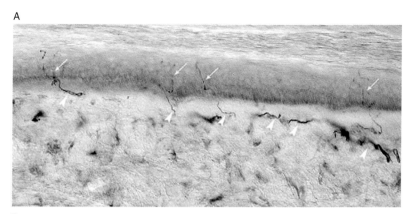

B

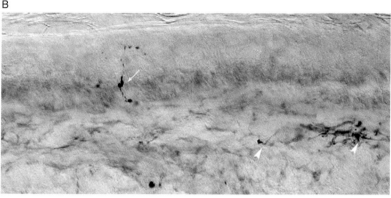

Figure 31.2. (A) Healthy control: normal density of intraepidermal nerve fibers ("small nerve fibers", arrows). Normal appearance of dermal nerve bundles (arrow heads). (B) Reduced number of intraepidermal nerve fibers in a patient with diabetic neuropathy. (From Sommer C, Lauria G. Skin biopsy in the management of peripheral neuropathy. *Lancet Neurol* 2007; **6**: 632–642, with permission.)

determined primarily by case history and physical examination. Small nerve fibers, thinly myelinated and unmyelinated, are often involved in patients with overt signs of a sensory or sensorimotor neuropathy. In these patients, needle EMG and nerve conduction studies help to establish the diagnosis. Electrophysiological examination, however, does not investigate small unmyelinated fibers and is typically normal in SFN. Denervation and reinnervation are signs of motor nerve dysfunction and are absent in SFN. Functional neurophysiological testing, including testing of autonomic function with heat sensitivity testing, for example, can provide relevant diagnostic information. These tests are not always easy to perform and require specific equipment that is not always available. A skin biopsy, on the other hand, is a validated technique for determining intraepidermal nerve fiber (IENF) density that can provide diagnostic, quantitative information if SFN is considered. Taking a skin biopsy is relatively easy and the procedure is relatively harmless. There is, however, a practical disadvantage of using a skin biopsy as a diagnostic tool, because determination of IENF density cannot be performed in most clinical laboratories.

There are various causes of SFN (Table 31.1). Frequently, no cause can be established. Especially in patients with I-SFN, the mechanisms that could lead to the signs and symptoms have remained obscure for a long period of time. Recent systematic genetic studies in patients meeting very strict criteria for I-SFN and biopsy confirmed I-SFN showed an almost 30% presence of gain-of-function mutations in the $Na_v1.7$ sodium channel (SCN9A) that is present on DRG and sympathetic ganglia and their small-diameter peripheral axons. Gain-of-function mutations can make these sodium channels hyperexcitable, leading to neuronal and length-dependent axonal degeneration and to clinical signs of painful SFN. This finding suggests an etiological basis for I-SFN. Prominent dysautonomia suggests SCN9A-related SFN.

Management of small fiber neuropathy depends on the underlying etiology with concurrent treatment of associated neuropathic pain. Pain due to SFN, however, is often difficult to treat. First of all, an underlying cause – when present – needs to be treated. If pain persists or when there is no probable underlying cause, treatment with antidepressants (like amitriptyline), anticonvulsants (such as pregabalin), opioids, topical therapies with capsaicin, or nonpharmacological treatments as part of the overall management of neuropathic pain can be tried. However, there is no best treatment for SFN, and most data are derived from studies that include patients with combined mixed neuropathic pain syndromes. Controlled trials studying the effect of pharmacological treatment of SFN are urgently needed.

Suggested reading

Devigili G, Tugnoli V, Penza P, et al. The diagnostic criteria for small fibre neuropathy: from symptoms to neuropathology. *Brain* 2008; **131**: 1912–1925.

England JD, Gronseth GS, Franklin G, et al. Practice parameter: the evaluation of distal symmetric polyneuropathy: the role of autonomic testing, nerve biopsy, and skin biopsy (an evidence-based review).

Report of the American Academy of Neurology, the American Association of Neuromuscular and Electrodiagnostic Medicine, and the American Academy of Physical Medicine and Rehabilitation. *Neurology* 2009; **72**: 177–184.

European Federation of Neurological Societies/Peripheral Nerve Society Guideline on the use of skin biopsy in the diagnosis of small fiber neuropathy. Report of a joint task force of the European Federation of Neurological Societies and the Peripheral Nerve Society. Joint Task Force of the EFNS and the PNS. *J Peripher Nerv Syst* 2010; **15**: 79–92.

Faber CG, Hoeijmakers JG, Ahn HS, et al. Gain of function Na$_v$1.7 mutations in idiopathic small fiber neuropathy. *Ann Neurol* 2012; **71**: 26–39.

Lauria G, Bakkers M, Schmitz C, et al. Intraepidermal nerve fiber density at the distal leg: a worldwide normative reference study. *J Peripher Nerv Syst* 2010; **15**: 202–207.

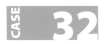

CASE 32 Critical illness polyneuropathy: a man who could not be weaned from the ventilator following evacuation of a cerebellar hematoma

Case history

A 64-year-old man with hypertension had acute-onset dysarthria and left-sided ataxia. A hematoma was diagnosed in the left cerebellar hemisphere. When he developed severe headaches and vertical gaze paresis, the neurosurgeon was consulted and a decision to evacuate the hematoma was made. After surgery, he developed pneumonia necessitating artificial ventilation. Further complications included metabolic alkalosis, sepsis, and hemodynamic instability. One week after surgery, he developed a tetraplegia.

Examination

He opened his eyes only after painful stimulation. Compression of the nail bed caused facial grimacing, which we interpreted as a localizing reaction following a painful stimulus. His eye movements were completely normal. His limbs were paralytic. After a few days, his best motor response was protrusion of the tongue on demand and blinking the eyes. He had flaccid tetraplegia with areflexia.

Ancillary investigations

Nine days after surgery, a brain MRI scan showed hypodensity within the left cerebellar hemisphere. The pons was normal and hydrocephalus was absent. CK activity and serum electrolyte concentrations were normal. After two weeks, needle EMG showed spontaneous muscle fiber activity in both anterior tibial muscles, but not in proximal leg muscles. Amplitudes of CMAPs of abductor pollicis brevis, abductor digiti quinti, and anterior tibial muscles were decreased. Distal motor latencies were normal. Sensory nerve action potentials were decreased.

Diagnostic considerations

In the process of differential diagnosis, the following disorders were considered, based on the clinical picture: locked-in syndrome, acute motor and sensory axonal neuropathy (a subtype of GBS) critical illness polyneuropathy (CIP), critical illness myopathy (CIM), acute myasthenia gravis, and acute myositis. The electrophysiological abnormalities suggested acute axonal sensory and motor polyneuropathy.

Follow-up

Complications were treated successfully. He received whole-body rehabilitation, consisting of interruption of sedation and physical and occupational therapy, after diagnosis of CIP. He could be weaned from the ventilator after eight weeks. He had developed severe skeletal muscle atrophy, distal more than proximal, and was transferred to a rehabilitation clinic. He was able to walk with a rollator after six months.

General remarks

CIP and CIM have, over the past 30 years, become increasingly recognized as complications of sepsis and multiorgan failure. CIP is the most frequent acute polyneuropathy encountered in the ICU. Patients

hospitalized in the ICU for more than one week are at risk. Essentially, they have limb weakness, usually diffuse, and cannot be weaned from the ventilator.

If CIP is suspected, other causes of diffuse weakness and difficult weaning must be excluded first. These include heart and lung disease, use of drugs that may block neuromuscular transmission or cause polyneuropathy, hypokalemia, hypophosphatemia, and hypocalcemia. Another explanation may be that the weakness is the first manifestation of myasthenia gravis. Very occasionally, patients with previously undiagnosed ALS or Pompe disease are admitted to the ICU with respiratory insufficiency during or following an attack of pneumonia. Differentiating CIP from acute motor and sensory axonal neuropathy can be cumbersome. The following factors can help in this

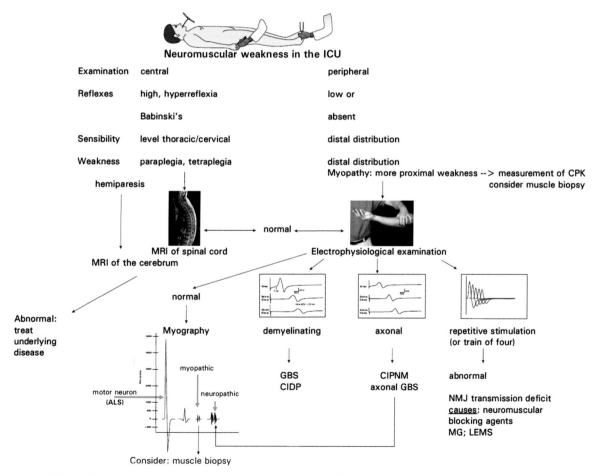

Figure 32.1. Algorithm for the approach to patients with muscle weakness in the intensive care unit. CIPNM, critical illness polyneuropathy and myopathy; NMJ, neuromuscular junction. Myopathic pattern: small amplitude and short-duration motor unit potentials; neuropathic pattern: polyphasic MUPs on needle EMG. (From Visser LH. Critical illness polyneuropathy and myopathy: clinical features, risk factors and prognosis. *Eur J Neurol* 2006; **13**: 1203–1211, with permission.)

A
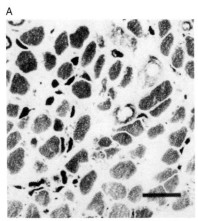

B
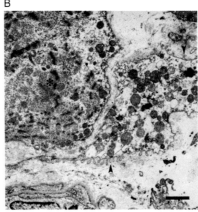

Figure 32.2. Critical illness myopathy. (A) Light microscopic section of intercostal muscle biopsy with type 2 muscle fiber atrophy (dark fibers). Atrophy of type 1 muscle fiber is less prominent (bar, 50 μm). (B) Electronmicrograph. No myofibrils are present in the atrophic muscle fiber at the right. Many basal lamina folds (arrowhead) confirm shrinkage of the muscle fiber. The fiber on the left shows the presence of some myofibrils and Z-disks (asterisk) (bar, 2 μm).

process. First, generally speaking, GBS is a reason for admission to the ICU; it does not develop in the ICU. Second, many patients will recall an antecedent infection. Third, facial muscles are frequently weak in GBS but not in CIP. Figure 32.1 presents a survey of the causes of neuromuscular weakness in the ICU.

CIM is a primary myopathy with distinctive electrophysiological and pathological features (Figure 32.2). The motor features of CIM and CIP are quite similar, hyporeflexia or areflexia occurring in both, but sensation should be normal in CIM. Electrophysiological tests may differentiate CIM from CIP because motor abnormalities prevail in CIM. CMAPs have decreased amplitude and increased duration, F-waves are absent, whereas SNAPs are normal. Needle EMG shows spontaneous muscle fiber activity and, if the patient is able to perform voluntary contraction, myopathic MUPs. During recovery, electrophysiological and pathological abnormalities in muscle will subside. Necrotizing ICU myopathy with myoglobinuria also forms part of the spectrum.

CIM should be differentiated from generalized skeletal muscle atrophy, which will usually become manifest after one to two weeks in severely ill or immobilized patients. They will be weak but not paralyzed and skeletal muscle biopsy will show predominantly type 2 muscle fiber atrophy. A similar catabolic event may occur following prolonged use of steroids (steroid myopathy). Recovery will be rapid once the patients become more active and well nourished or after gradual cessation of steroids.

The cause of CIP and CIM has not yet been identified. A multifactorial origin is likely, involving microcirculatory, cellular, and metabolic pathophysiological factors. Onset of clinical signs can be rapid, and initially,

the electrophysiological abnormalities may be reversible. CIP and CIM can cause prolonged and severe disability. It has been estimated that about one-third of patients who survive will no longer be able to walk independently or breathe spontaneously. Patients with CIM may have a better prognosis than those with CIP, confirming the general notion in neurology of a difficult recovery following axonal degeneration of peripheral nerves once the cause of the neuropathy has been treated successfully.

No specific treatments exist, but the importance of supportive measures is being recognized increasingly. These include prevention of pressure palsies, and early rehabilitation in the ICU. A protocol of coordinated daily interruption of sedatives with spontaneous awakening and interruption of mechanical ventilation with spontaneous breathing trials may reduce the duration of mechanical ventilation, coma, and ICU and hospital stay. More ventilator-free days compared with standard care, a shorter duration of delirium, and better functional outcomes at hospital discharge has been achieved with early physical and occupational therapy.

Suggested reading

Girard TD, Kreis JP, Fuchs BD, et al. Efficacy and safety of a paired sedation and ventilator weaning protocol for mechanical ventilated patients in intensive care (Awakening and Breathing Controlled trial): a randomised controlled trial. *Lancet* 2008; **371**: 126–134.

Guarneri B, Bertolini G, Latronico N. Long-term outcome in patients with critical illness myopathy or neuropathy: the Italian multicentre CRIMYNE study. *J Neurol Neurosurg Psychiatry* 2008; **79**: 838–841.

Latronico N, Bolton CF. Critical illness polyneuropathy and myopathy: a major cause of muscle weakness and paralysis. *Lancet Neurol* 2011; **10**: 931–941.

Schweickert WD, Pohlman MC, Pohlman AS, et al. Early physical and occupational therapy in mechanically

ventilated, critically ill patients: a randomised controlled trial. *Lancet* 2009; **373**: 1874–1882.

Visser LH. Critical illness polyneuropathy and myopathy: clinical features, risk factors and prognosis. *Eur J Neurol* 2006; **13**: 1203–1211.

CASE 33

Chronic idiopathic axonal polyneuropathy: a man, unsteady on his legs, who had to buy a new car

Clinical history

A 62-year-old man complained of unsteadiness when walking and numbness on the soles of both feet. He was unsteady when washing his hair under the shower. On uneven surfaces, he had to take care not to stumble. He had to buy a car with automatic transmission because of difficulties operating the brake and accelerator pedals.

For about 10 years, he had experienced tingling sensations in the left toes that spread to the right side, and over the years, gradually moved upward to halfway up the lower legs. He experienced a stiff feeling in the feet and lower legs and frequent nightly cramps in both calves, but no pain. For the past year, he complained about numb fingertips with some loss of dexterity. He did not have dry eyes or mouth. He did not use vitamins or drugs and alcohol intake was sparse. The family history was not informative.

Examination

We only found weakness of his toe extensor muscles, MRC grade 4. Vibration sense was decreased in the middle fingers and absent in the toes and halfway up his feet. Movement sense in the toes was decreased. Pain and tactile sense were abnormal at the fingertips and below the knees, but sharp–dull discrimination was normal. The Achilles tendon reflexes were absent. After walking a short distance, he developed bilateral foot drop.

Ancillary investigations

Previously, another neurologist had detected no metabolic abnormalities and no vitamin deficiency. We found no abnormalities to indicate an immune-mediated disease (Table 33.1). Needle EMG showed mild spontaneous muscle fiber activity and neurogenic

MUPs in the left foot extensor muscles, minor slowing of nerve conduction velocity, and decreased SNAPs. These findings suggested mild axonal polyneuropathy.

Diagnostic considerations

A diagnosis of chronic idiopathic axonal polyneuropathy (CIAP) with predominant sensory symptoms and signs was made. The absence of affected family members virtually excludes CMT type 2. The long disease history excludes paraneoplastic neuropathy.

General remarks

In a patient with a clinical diagnosis of sensory and motor polyneuropathy and negative family history, a step-wise diagnostic course is advised. The first step is to exclude diabetes mellitus, alcohol abuse, or renal insufficuency. Careful evaluation with the patient in a supine position can reveal whether there is pes cavus suggesting CMT disease. If diabetes is found in a patient with a mainly sensory stocking-and-glove neuropathy, no additional tests are necessary to confirm the diagnosis of neuropathy (Case 24).

If diabetes is absent, the second step is electrophysiological assessment, which should:

1. Confirm the presence of neuropathy. Pure motor abnormalities must lead to revision of the diagnosis. ALS, PMA, and also sIBM are alternative explanations in some patients.
2. Detect abnormalities in arm nerves. Usually these are less prominent compared with abnormalities of leg nerves. If only motor abnormalities in leg nerves are found, spinal dural arteriovenous fistula or multiple radiculopathies can be the explanation.
3. Differentiate between axonal and demyelinating neuropathy (Cases 9 and 16).

Table 33.1. Diagnosis that must be considered in the analysis of axonal sensory or sensory and motor polyneuropathy

Disease	Appropriate tests
Diabetes mellitus	Fasting glucose and glycolysated hemoglobin (HbA1c)
Renal insufficiency[a]	Creatinine, ureum
Alcoholism	γ-glutamyl tranferase (GGT), alanine aminotransferase (ALAT)
Hypothyroidism	TSH
Vitamin B1 deficiency	Thiamine (B1)
Vitamin B6 deficiency[b]	Pyridoxine (B6)
Vitamin B6 intoxication[b]	B6
Vitamin B12 deficiency[c]	Cyanocobalamin (B12), fasting plasma homocysteine, plasma methylmalonic acid
Monoclonal gammopathy	Serum and urine M-protein electrophoresis and immunofixation, free light chains
Sjögren syndrome	ANA, line-blot ENA
Malignancy[d]	ANNA-1 and other antineuronal antibodies

[a] Neuropathy not an early sign, motor signs predominate
[b] Ataxic signs predominate
[c] Neuropathy can be the only manifestation of vitamin B12 (cobalamin) deficiency. Normal or low serum cobalamin levels can be associated with abnormal serum metabolite concentrations (methylmalonic acid and homocysteine), suggestive of cobalamine deficiency. Autoimmune pernicious anemia can be diagnosed in some of these patients with normal serum cobalamine levels. Not all patients with cobalamin deficiency show concomitant pyramidal signs (combined tract degeneration)
[d] Paraneoplastic neuropathy: rapid progression (weeks–months, sensory and ataxic signs predominate, may precede tumor signs by one year (Case 22)

Table 33.2. Characteristic features of chronic idiopathic axonal polyneuropathy

Onset	After age 50 years
Site of onset	Toes, soles of feet, can start asymmetrically
Clinical features	Sensory or sensory and motor, not purely motor
Male:female ratio	2:1
Progression	Slow (months–years)
Pain in the feet	Can be present and incapacitating
Weakness of distal leg muscles	2/3 of patients
Claw toes, pes cavus	Rare
Weakness of hand muscles	1/6 of patients
CK elevation (rarely >2 x ULN)	<5%
Walking aids[a]	1/4 of patients
Autonomic signs	Absent[b]

[a] Walking aids: cane, adjusted shoes, ankle–foot orthosis, rollator (wheeled walker) in patients >65 years old
[b] If autonomic signs are evident, consider again diabetes, monoclonal gammopathy with primary amyloidosis, and familial amyloid polyneuropathy with mutation in the transthyretrin gene

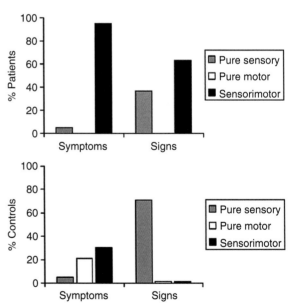

Figure 33.1. Symptoms and signs of patients with CIAP (upper panel) and control subjects (lower panel), for pure sensory (gray shaded bars), pure motor (open bars), and sensorimotor (solid bars) functions. (From Vrancken AF, Franssen H, Wokke JH, et al. Chronic idiopathic axonal polyneuropathy and successful aging of the peripheral nervous system in elderly people. *Arch Neurol* 2002; **59**: 533–540, with permission.)

If EMG suggests sensory and motor axonal neuropathy, the third step is an extensive search for metabolic disturbances, vitamin deficiency and autoimmune dysregulation (Table 33.1).

CIAP is a diagnosis by exclusion in 10%–20% of patients with neuropathy (Table 33.2). Pain suggests involvement of small nerve fibers. Some patients cannot tolerate wearing socks. If motor symptoms predominate, a diagnosis of late-onset CMT type 2 should be considered. Usually, patients remain ambulant and wheelchair dependency does not occur.

The cause of CIAP is probably heterogeneous. No association with alcohol, venous insufficiency, peripheral arterial disease, or antibodies to peripheral antigens have been found. Signs suggestive of polyneuropathy occur with increasing age in healthy persons, probably due to aging of the nervous system. These signs are predominantly sensory and include loss of light touch sense, vibration sense at the toes and feet, and Achilles jerks. Compared with age-matched, healthy persons, patients with CIAP have more signs (Figure 33.1). There is no effective treatment for CIAP. Treatment of pain is symptomatic.

Suggested reading

Benson MD, Kincaid JC. The molecular biology and clinical features of amyloid neuropathy. *Muscle Nerve* 2007; **36**: 411–423.

Hughes RAC, Umapathi T, Gray IA, et al. A controlled investigation of the cause of chronic idiopathic axonal polyneuropathy. *Brain* 2004; **127**: 1723–1730.

Saperstein DS, Wolfe GI, Gronseth GS, et al. Challenges in the identification of cobalamin-deficiency polyneuropathy. *Arch Neurol* 2003; **60**: 1296–1301.

Teunissen LL, Notermans NC, Franssen H, et al. Differences between hereditary motor and sensory neuropathy type 2 and chronic idiopathic axonal neuropathy. A clinical and electrophysiological study. *Brain* 1997; **120**: 955–962.

Vrancken AFJE, Franssen H, Wokke JHJ, Teunissen LT, Notermans NC. Chronic idiopathic axonal polyneuropathy and successful aging of the peripheral nervous system in elderly people. *Arch Neurol* 2002; **59**: 533–540.

CASE 34

Classic myasthenia gravis: an elderly woman with impaired speech following abdominal surgery

Clinical history

A 70-year-old woman was referred by her GP because of progressive nasal speech and difficulties with chewing and swallowing, shortly after undergoing abdominal surgery three months earlier because of a "borderline" malignant cystoadenofibroma of the uterus. Weeks later, she also noticed drooping of both eyelids and a tendency for her head to drop at the end of a day. In retrospect, slightly nasal speech had been present for some months prior to surgery.

Examination

VC was normal for age and height. An asymmetric ptosis at inspection increased after looking upward for 20 s, with the eyelid closing down on the pupil. She had no diplopia. There was a mild bulbar dysarthria and mild weakness of neck extensor muscles. Atrophy and fasciculation of the tongue were absent.

Ancillary investigations

The level of serum acetylcholine receptor (AChR) autoantibodies was increased and autoantibodies to striated muscle proteins were detectable. CT scanning of the chest showed signs of a thymoma measuring 1.4 in × 1.1 in.

Diagnostic considerations

Both the clinical history and the neurological examination provided evidence of fluctuating muscle weakness. The clinical diagnosis of myasthenia gravis was confirmed swiftly, by the finding of an increased level of serum AChR autoantibodies. Because of the age at presentation, bulbar onset, and the finding of a thymoma and autoantibodies to striated muscle proteins, it was stressed to the patient that she should be extra alert and report any worsening promptly because she was considered to be at risk of rapid respiratory failure.

Follow-up

Pyridostigmine had no effect and bulbar weakness worsened over days. She improved quickly on high-dose prednisolone (1 mg/kg/d). Azathioprine was not well tolerated. Thymoma surgery was followed by gradual improvement. In subsequent years, she had several periods of increased bulbar weakness when under physical or emotional stress. These were successfully treated with an increase in prednisolone dose or with IVIg. Seven years after presentation she had surgery for a colon carcinoma.

A

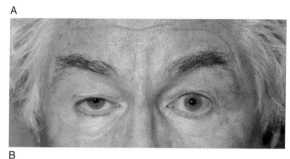

B

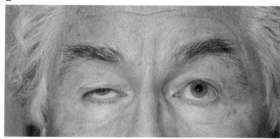

C

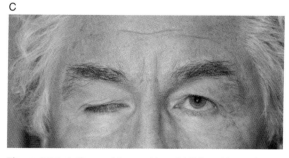

Figure 34.1. A 62-year-old man with anti-AChR-positive ocular myasthenia gravis. (A–C) Right-sided slight ptosis at rest, worsening to almost complete ptosis, and slight left-sided ptosis in the course of looking up for 30 seconds.

Table 34.1. Provocation tests when myasthenia gravis is suspected

- Diplopia: ask the patient to look upward or sideways for one minute
- Ptosis: observe whether ptosis occurs while looking upwards for one minute. Ptosis can be asymmetric. Stop when the falling eyelid covers the pupil
- During the same procedure, the strength of the neck muscles can be tested before and after looking upward for one minute
- The occurrence of dysarthria
- Total of numbers added up while counted aloud during one breath
- Number of seconds that the arms can be stretched out while in the sitting position. Measure strength of the deltoid muscles, using the MRC scale, before and after stretching out. Stop after one minute of stretching out.
- Number of seconds that legs can be straightened in the supine position
- Number of times able to stand up from squatting position (stop at 10)

Table 34.2. Neostigmine test

- Inform the patient about the test and the possible side effects
- Start with 0.5 mg atropine SC or IM (to prevent side effects of neostigmine)
- After five minutes: specific provocation tests depending on localization of weakness (Table 34.1). This part of the protocol can be used to test for a possible placebo effect
- After the examination: administer 1.5 mg neostigmine SC or IM
- Repeat specific provocation tests after five and 10 minutes, and if no improvement is observed, repeat after 15, 20, and 30 minutes
- Observe the patient for at least 30 minutes after neostigmine administration for possible side effects (decreased heart rate, gastrointestinal symptoms, e.g., diarrhoea)
- Neostigmine test is considered to be positive if there is no improvement of the functional tests after atropine and when there is a clearly positive response after neostigmine administration

During the ensuing years, myasthenia gravis remained stable on low-dose prednisolone.

General remarks

Of all acquired disorders of the neuromuscular junction, myasthenia gravis caused by IgG-autoantibodies directed toward the skeletal muscle AChR is the most common. About 85% of patients with generalized myasthenia gravis have these antibodies. The clinical hallmark is weakness of specific muscles, which is aggravated by activity of these muscles and improves with rest. Fluctuating, asymmetric external ophthalmoplegia is the most frequent presentation (Figure 34.1; Video 16). The disease may remain confined to extraocular weakness, but generalized weakness usually develops within two years. If onset is in young adulthood (<40 yr), patients are most frequently female. Spontaneous long-lasting remission occurs occasionally in this group. In older patients, the frequent finding of antibodies to striated muscle proteins, such as titin, the ryanodine-receptor, and voltage-gated K channel alpha subunit, Kv1.4, is associated with more severe disease with oropharyngeal weakness and myasthenic crises, and also with a thymoma. Isolated myasthenic bulbar weakness in younger women is more likely to be caused by anti-MuSK than anti-AChR antibodies (Case 35).

If myasthenia gravis is suspected, provocation tests (Table 34.1), and the neostigmine test (Table 34.2) may be of diagnostic value. An increased level of serum antibody to muscle AChR definitely confirms the diagnosis of classic myasthenia gravis in a patient with a typical clinical presentation, but test results are only available after some weeks.

Useful electrophysiological tests include repetitive 3 Hz nerve stimulation of the ulnar, accessory, and facial nerves, showing a decremental response of the CMAP in a symptomatic muscle (Figure 34.2). Single-fiber EMG is particularly useful in diagnosing ocular myasthenia gravis. Antibody tests and EMG have high sensitivity and specificity in generalized myasthenia gravis. The neostigmine test gives immediate results, but may be difficult to interpret (Table 34.2). Imaging of the chest to search for a thymoma should be performed in all patients. Rarely, a malignant thymoma can be detected.

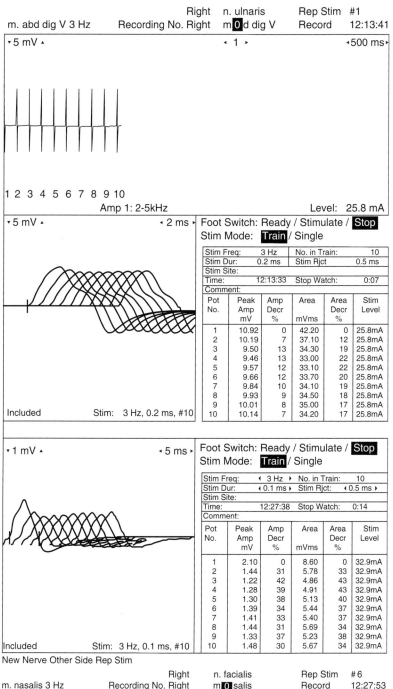

Right n. ulnaris Rep Stim #1
m. abd dig V 3 Hz   Recording No. Right   m**0**d dig V   Record   12:13:41

Pot No.	Peak Amp mV	Amp Decr %	Area mVms	Area Decr %	Stim Level
1	10.92	0	42.20	0	25.8mA
2	10.19	7	37.10	12	25.8mA
3	9.50	13	34.30	19	25.8mA
4	9.46	13	33.00	22	25.8mA
5	9.57	12	33.10	22	25.8mA
6	9.66	12	33.70	20	25.8mA
7	9.84	10	34.10	19	25.8mA
8	9.93	9	34.50	18	25.8mA
9	10.01	8	35.00	17	25.8mA
10	10.14	7	34.20	17	25.8mA

Foot Switch: Ready / Stimulate / Stop
Stim Mode: Train / Single

Stim Freq:	3 Hz	No. in Train:	10
Stim Dur:	0.2 ms	Stim Rjct	0.5 ms
Stim Site:			
Time:	12:13:33	Stop Watch:	0:07
Comment:			

Included   Stim: 3 Hz, 0.2 ms, #10

Pot No.	Peak Amp mV	Amp Decr %	Area mVms	Area Decr %	Stim Level
1	2.10	0	8.60	0	32.9mA
2	1.44	31	5.78	33	32.9mA
3	1.22	42	4.86	43	32.9mA
4	1.28	39	4.91	43	32.9mA
5	1.30	38	5.13	40	32.9mA
6	1.39	34	5.44	37	32.9mA
7	1.41	33	5.40	37	32.9mA
8	1.44	31	5.69	34	32.9mA
9	1.33	37	5.23	38	32.9mA
10	1.48	30	5.67	34	32.9mA

Foot Switch: Ready / Stimulate / Stop
Stim Mode: Train / Single

Stim Freq:	◄ 3 Hz ►	No. in Train:	10
Stim Dur:	◄ 0.1 ms ►	Stim Rjct	◄ 0.5 ms ►
Stim Site:			
Time:	12:27:38	Stop Watch:	0:14
Comment:			

Included   Stim: 3 Hz, 0.1 ms, #10

New Nerve Other Side Rep Stim

Right n. facialis Rep Stim #6
m. nasalis 3 Hz   Recording No. Right   m**0**salis   Record   12:27:53

Figure 34.2. Decrement of the CMAP during 3 Hz nerve stimulation in a patient with myasthenia gravis. As typical in classic myasthenia gravis, each decrement is U-shaped: the CMAP-decrease is most prominent with the fourth or fifth stimulus. Thereafter the decremental response becomes less pronounced. Upper and middle panels: stimulation of the ulnar nerve at the wrist with recording from abductor digiti minimi muscle shows a decrement of up to 13%. Lower panel: stimulation of a facial nerve branch at the cheek with recording from the nasal muscle shows a decrement of up to 42%.

The treatment of first choice is a cholinesterase inhibitor (pyridostigmine) in sufficiently high and frequent doses. Most patients need 6 × 60 mg/d; some need a controlled release form of the drug before the night. Diarrhea, salivation, and bronchorrhea are parasympathetic side effects of pyridostigmine that usually disappear spontaneously after a few weeks. Cramps and fasciculation may also occur (Video 3). Persisting or severe parasympathetic side effects can be treated with atropine sulphate 0.125–0.25 mg per dose of pyridostigmine.

AChR antibody-positive, early onset patients with generalized myasthenia gravis and insufficient response to pyridostigmine therapy should be considered for thymectomy, although hard evidence of efficacy of thymectomy is missing. Thymomas should always be surgically removed because of the dangers of infiltrative growth. If the effect of pyridostigmine is not satisfactory, the benefits of prednisolone (1–1.5 mg/kg) together with azathioprine (2–3 × 50 mg/d) should be weighed against the adverse effects with long-term use. There is no consensus whether patients with generalized myasthenia gravis should be admitted at instalment of corticosteroid treatment. Further deterioration with prednisolone has been observed. High-dose prednisolone is administered for four to six weeks. Some advocate starting with low dose (20 mg daily) prednisolone and building up in weeks. After this period, the dosage can be tapered gradually to a maintenance therapy of 15–25 mg on alternate days, for example. Once stabilization has been achieved and the patient has recovered, further tapering can be tried. Some patients are kept on azathioprine for years. Anti-AChR antibody titers may decrease, but some patients in remission maintain high titers. With treatment, many patients will be able to return to work and be socially active.

About 50% of patients with ocular myasthenia gravis have anti-AChR antibodies. At present, it is not possible to make evidence-based recommendations regarding the effects of cholinesterase inhibitors, corticosteroids, or other immunosuppressive agents with respect to pure ocular symptoms. We start with cholinesterase inhibitors, and if these have no effect, add low doses of prednisolone (20–40 mg daily).

A relapse can occur, sometimes after many years. Anti-AChR antibodies mediate complement-induced destruction of the postsynaptic endplate region. New endplates will develop on the muscle nearby (Figure 34.3), but this regenerative process may fail in elderly or severely affected patients. Patients who have myasthenia gravis for a long period of time may, therefore, develop residual atrophy of muscles. Atrophy can affect bulbar muscles (See Introduction, Figure 4), but also limb muscles, like the deltoid muscle. Older patients with bulbar weakness or weak respiratory muscles, as well as their doctor, should be especially aware of the possibility of acute and rapid deterioration resulting in life-threatening respiratory weakness. Acute exacerbation of myasthenia gravis with severe bulbar, respiratory, or generalized symptoms, myasthenic crisis, is treated with PE or IVIg with similar efficacy and complication rates. Patients with classic myasthemia gravis who receive general anesthesia for surgery may have difficulties with weaning from the ventilator. The anesthesiologist should be informed about the diagnosis.

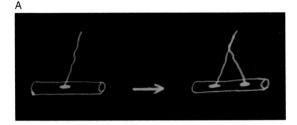

Figure 34.3. Normally one muscle fiber has a single endplate area (A). Anti-AChR antibodies induce destruction of endplates through activation of complement. As a repair mechanism, new endplate regions of even whole endplates will develop nearby destructed ones. (B) (myasthenia gravis): lower muscle fiber has two end plates with one newly induced by a preterminal nerve sprout. Nuclei and endplate regions are stained dark (silver-cholinesterase staining).

Suggested reading

Benatar M, Kaminski HJ. Practice parameter: the medical treatment of ocular myasthenia (an evidence-based review). Report of the Quality Standards Subcommittee of the American Academy of Neurology. *Neurology* 2007; **68**: 2144–2149.

Mandawat A, Kaminski HJ, Cutter G, Katjiri B, Alshekhlee A. Comparitive analysis of therapeutic options used for myasthenia gravis. *Ann Neurol* 2010; **68**: 797–805.

Meriggioli MN, Sanders DB. Autoimmune myasthenia gravis: emerging clinical and biological heterogeneity. *Lancet Neurol* 2009; **8**: 475–490.

Saperstein DS, Barohn RJ. Management of myasthenia gravis. *Semin Neurol* 2004; **24**: 41–48.

Skeie GO, Apostolski S, Evoli A, et al. Guidelines for treatment of autoimmune neuromuscular transmission disorders. *Eur J Neurol* 2010; **17**: 893–902.

Verschuuren JJGM, Palace J, Gilhus NE. Clinical aspects of myasthenia explained. *Autoimmunity* 2010; **43**: 344–352.

Vincent A. Autoimmune mediated neuromuscular junction defects. *Curr Opin Neurol* 2010; **23**: 489–495.

Myasthenia gravis with autoantibodies to muscle-specific kinase: a woman who could not lift her arms following abdominal surgery

Clinical history

Over a period of months, a 45-year-old woman noticed that she could not raise her arms well. She also reported double vision in the evening that, in retrospect, had been present for some years. Three years later, it became difficult for her to keep her head up without support, to chew, and to swallow, which sometimes worsened for weeks at a time.

Examination

There was asymmetric diplopia after 15 seconds of gazing sideways, mild weakness of neck extensor and flexor muscles, and weak shoulder abduction. Speech and respiration were normal.

Ancillary investigations

EMG showed a pathological (20%) decrement on 3 Hz stimulation of the nasal and trapezius muscles that confirmed a defect of postsynaptic neuromuscular transmission in these muscles. On single fiber EMG of the orbicularis oculi muscle, an abnormal jitter was noted. Autoantibodies to AChR were not detected, excluding classic myasthenia gravis (Case 34). Autoantibodies to muscle-specific kinase (MuSK) were present.

Diagnostic considerations

Diplopia and bulbar symptoms and signs that vary in intensity are suggestive of myasthenia gravis. Electrophysiological tests confirmed the presence of a postsynaptic transmission disorder. Bulbar signs are common in anti-MuSK myasthenia gravis, and diplopia and ptosis may be present early in the disease. Myasthenia gravis occasionally becomes manifest following stressful events such as surgery.

Follow-up

During subsequent years, weakness progressed. For symptomatic treatment she received pyridostigmine with little effect. During the course of the disease, she was treated with prednisolone (and osteoporosis prophylaxis), azathioprine, IVIg, and mycophenolate mofetil. Fifteen years after presentation, she receives immunosuppression with prednisolone 15 mg and azathioprine 100 mg daily. The myasthenic symptoms are reasonably

A

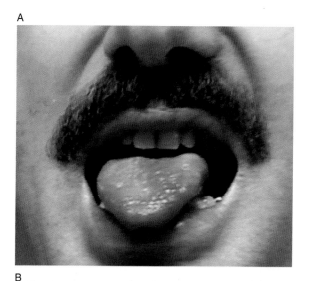

B

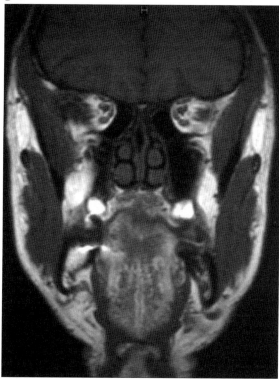

Figure 35.1. Atrophy of the tongue in a man with anti-MuSK myasthenia gravis (A). Note the vertical position of the nasolabial folds. T-1 weighted MRI scan shows replacement of the tongue muscle by fat (B). (Courtesy of Professor Jan Verschuuren.)

107

well controlled. In addition, she was treated for the prednisolone-related side effects of hypertension, diabetes mellitus, and gastric complaints.

General remarks

About 15% of patients with generalized myasthenia gravis do not have detectable anti-AChR antibodies. It has been estimated that about 40% of these patients have anti-MuSK antibodies. MuSK is a transmembrane endplate polypeptide involved in maintenance of the high-density AChR clustering at the muscle endplate. Anti-MuSK myasthenia gravis is typically diagnosed in young women. EMG with repetitive nerve stimulation and the edrophonium test are less sensitive than in anti-AChR myasthenia gravis. More often than in anti-AChR myasthenia gravis, weakness is facial and bulbar. Marked atrophy can be observed; of the tongue, for example (Figure 35.1). Respiratory crises are more common. The response to pyridostigmine is less evident than in anti-AChR myasthenia gravis. Some patients do not even tolerate pyridostigmine. Thymus hyperplasia or thymoma are usually not found, and it is not clear whether thymectomy is indicated in these patients. Rituximab may have a long-lasting beneficial effect in anti-MuSK myasthenia gravis, with decrease in antibody titers.

Suggested reading

Diaz-Manera J, Martinez-Hernandez E, Querol L, et al. Long-lasting treatment effect of rituximab in MuSK myasthenia. *Neurology* 2012; **78**: 189–193.

Guptill JT, Sanders DB. Update on muscle-specific tyrosine kinase antibody positive myasthenia gravis. *Curr Opin Neurol* 2010; **23**: 530–535.

Pasnoor M, Wolfe GI, Nations S, et al. Clinical findings in MuSK-antibody positive myasthenia gravis: a U.S. experience. *Muscle Nerve* 2010; **41**: 370–374.

Skeie GO, Apostolski S, Evoli A, et al. Guidelines for treatment of autoimmune neuromuscular transmission disorders. *Eur J Neurol* 2010; **17**: 893–902.

Verschuuren JJGM, Palace J, Gilhus NE. Clinical aspects of myasthenia explained. *Autoimmunity* 2010; **43**: 344–352.

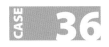

Lambert–Eaton myasthenic syndrome: a woman who smoked heavily and who could not walk anymore

Clinical history

A 33-year-old woman, who several years ago was diagnosed with chronic fatigue syndrome, noticed a lead-like feeling and progressive weakness in her upper legs over a period of four months. Climbing stairs became very difficult, and eventually she could no longer walk independently. She had no symptoms in her arms. There were no sensory symptoms. During this period, it became obvious that her voice changed; it seemed as though she were speaking "like a drunk", especially if she were tired. There were no complaints about double vision, a drooping eyelid, or swallowing. She did not drink alcohol, but had smoked at least a pack of cigarettes per day for many years.

Examination

The patient was sitting in a wheelchair, could barely stand, and could only walk with help. She had a bulbar dysarthria. She had ptosis that increased somewhat after looking upward, but no diplopia. There was mild weakness of the neck flexor muscles. Overt skel-

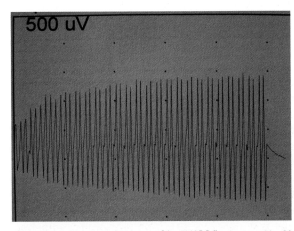

Figure 36.1. Incremental response of the CMAP following repetitive 20 Hz nerve stimulation. The amplitude of the initial action potential is too low (500 μV). The following amplitudes increase gradually to a normal value.

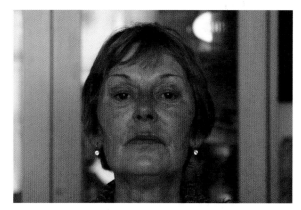

Figure 36.2. Mild ptosis in a patient with LEMS and SCLC.

etal muscle atrophy and fasciculation were absent. She had a symmetric paresis of the arms – proximal more than distal – MRC grade 4. The proximal muscles of the legs were severely paretic (MRC grade 2), with distal weakness (MRC grade 4). There were no sensory disturbances. The muscle tendon reflexes were reduced. Interestingly, repetitive movements against force induced a clear improvement in weakness of arms and legs.

Ancillary investigations and diagnostic considerations

The patient presented with limb girdle pattern weakness, but from the clinical examination, a neuromuscular transmission disorder was likely. Therefore, we did a neostigmine test (see Table 34.2) that showed a spectacular increase in muscle strength. She could even stand and walk unaided after the test. We started pyridostigmine treatment (3 × 40 mg/d) and tested for antibodies to AChRs, as some patients with classic myasthenia gravis present with limb girdle weakness. As a presynaptic disorder of neuromuscular transmission was suggested from the observation of increased strength following repetitive movement, and as she was a heavy smoker, antibodies against voltage-gated calcium channels (VGCC) were also determined. The test for anti-AChR antibodies was negative, but anti-VGCC antibodies were found.

After stopping pyridostigmine, EMG was performed. CMAPs had low amplitudes. Repetitive 20 Hz nerve stimulation revealed a clear increase in CMAPs, compatible with the Lambert–Eaton myasthenic syndrome (LEMS; Figure 36.1).

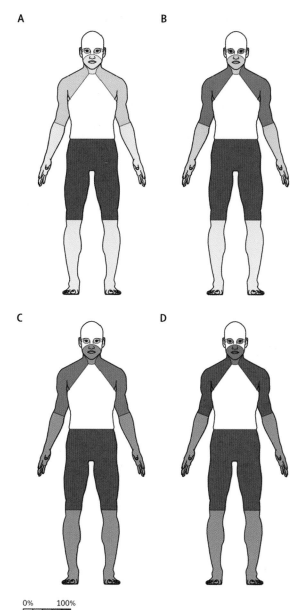

Figure 36.3. Spreading of symptoms in patients with nontumor (NT)-associated LEMS and SCLC–LEMS. Frequency of symptoms at three months (A) and 12 months (B) in patients with NT–LEMS, and frequency of symptoms at three months (C) and 12 months (D) in patients with SCLC–LEMS. The percentages describe the approximate proportion of patients who have that symptom within the given timeframe. (From Titulaer MJ, Lang B, Verschuuren JJGM. Lambert–Eaton myasthenic syndrome: from clinical characteristics to therapeutic strategies. *Lancet Neurol* 2011; **10**: 1098–1107, with permission.)

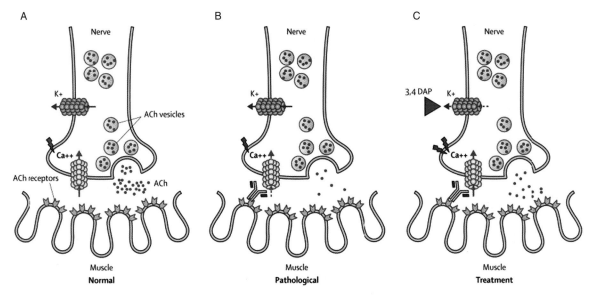

Figure 36.4. Pathophysiology of LEMS and effects of symptomatic treatment. (A) Normal depolarization of the presynaptic nerve terminal leading to ACh release, and ultimately, muscle contraction. (B) In LEMS, antibodies against VGCC block calcium influx leading to reduced ACh release. (C) Treatment with 3,4-diaminopyridine (red triangles) blocks efflux of potassium ions, prolonging the duration of depolarization. This keeps the pathologically affected calcium channels open longer, which leads to increased ability of the ACh vesicles to fuse and release neurotransmitter. (From Titulaer MJ, Lang B, Verschuuren JJGM. Lambert–Eaton myasthenic syndrome: from clinical characteristics to therapeutic strategies. *Lancet Neurol* 2011; **10**: 1098–1107, with permission.)

Follow-up

Once it became evident that she had LEMS after smoking heavily for many years, the lungs were the target of further investigations. Pulmonary investigations revealed that she had small-cell lung cancer (SCLC). She was treated with cytostatics. Unfortunately, an increase in pyridostigmine did not result in further improvement of muscle weakness. Treatment with 3,4 diaminopyridine was started and resulted in improved muscle strength. Time will reveal whether cytostatic treatment of her SCLC has a therapeutic effect.

General remarks

LEMS is a neuromuscular autoimmune disease, frequently associated with a malignancy, most often SCLC. In LEMS, characteristic muscle weakness is thought to be caused by pathogenic autoantibodies directed against VGCC that are present on the presynaptic nerve terminal. SLCC also expresses functional VGCC. VGCC play an important role in the release of acetylcholine from the nerve terminals at the neuromuscular junction following nerve stimulation during normal activity and at stimulation during EMG. In patients with LEMS, the function of VGCC is blocked by these antibodies. Sustained muscle activity and

high-frequency electrical nerve stimulation both prevent outward flow of Ca^{2+}-ions, resulting in increased availability of Ca^{2+}-ions in terminal axon branches. The latter will increase the likelihood of presynaptic acetylcholine release so that both muscle strength and CMAPs increase.

However, not all LEMS patients have a tumor. In these patients, LEMS is considered to be primary autoimmune in nature. Patients with nonmalignant LEMS may be treated for a couple of months or – more likely – years, whereafter they can be completely symptom free even after tapering of the medication. Of all LEMS patients with or without malignancy, 85% have antibodies to VGCC.

The clinical triad of LEMS typically consists of proximal muscle weakness, autonomic features, and areflexia. The initial symptom in most patients is proximal leg weakness that spreads rapidly to the proximal arm and shoulder muscles, and next to distal muscles and to the oculobulbar region. Patients with LEMS associated with SCLC have more rapid progression. Mild ptosis may occur (Figure 36.2). In contrast to classic myasthenia gravis, isolated ophthalmoplegia is rare (Figure 36.3).

Despite the fact that a neostigmine test can be clearly positive and can help in reaching the diagnosis, maintenance treatment with pyridostigmine is much less effective than in patients with myasthenia gravis.

Using a scoring system, the chance of a LEMS patient having SCLC can easily be determined. Age at onset, smoking behavior, weight loss, Karnofsky score, bulbar involvement, male sexual impotence, and the presence of Sry-like high-mobility group box protein 1 (SOX) serum antibodies are independent predictors for SCLC in LEMS. For SCLC–LEMS, tumor therapy is essential. In all patients with LEMS, targeted symptomatic therapy is 3,4 di-aminopyridine (Figure 36.4). Immunosuppression can also be of help.

Suggested reading

Keogh M, Sedehizadeh S, Maddison P. Treatment for Lambert–Eaton myasthenic syndrome. *Cochrane Database Syst Rev* 2011; CD003279.

Titulaer MJ, Lang B, Verschuuren JJ. Lambert-Eaton myasthenic syndrome: from clinical characteristics to therapeutic strategies. *Lancet Neurol* 2011; **10**: 1098–1107.

Titulaer MJ, Maddison P, Sont JK, et al. Clinical Dutch–English Lambert–Eaton myasthenic syndrome (LEMS) tumor association prediction score accurately predicts small-cell lung cancer in the LEMS. *J Clin Oncol* 2011; **29**: 902–908.

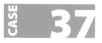

37 Congenital myasthenic syndrome, slow channel syndrome: a nurse with drooping eyelids and limb weakness

Clinical history

A 21-year-old nurse experienced problems when she had to grip objects firmly. She had to give up her work as a nurse. From the age of 16 years, drooping of the eyelids and a change in facial expression were noted by her family. She could never keep up with peers at sports and was unable to raise herself by her arms at gymnastics. At the age of 23 years, she developed weakness of the legs.

Examination

Three years after onset, she had a ptosis of about 25% that increased on lateral gaze. She lacked facial expression. The temporal muscle was well developed and skeletal muscle atrophy was absent. Neck flexor and extensor muscles were weak, MRC grade 4–5. After a period of rest, the initial strength of most other muscles was normal but weakness developed rapidly on provocation (Case 34; see Table 34.1). When walking, she developed a waddling gait. Walking on heels and toes was only possible for three steps.

Ancillary investigations and diagnostic considerations

Myasthenia gravis was considered, but weakness increased with anticholinesterase drugs and antibodies to AChR were absent. After repetitive stimulation with 3 Hz, there was a 15%–40% decrement of the CMAPs in abductor digit quinti, abductor pollicis brevis, and deltoid muscles. There was a double CMAP to single stimuli and to the first stimulus during repetitive stimulation (Figure 37.1). The second repetitive response occurred 7–10 msec after the first and its amplitude was always smaller. Endplate studies in intact isolated muscle fibers showed prolonged decay times of miniature endplate potentials and severe destruction of postsynaptic areas and of subendplate muscle (Figure 37.2).

Follow-up

In subsequent years, her condition stabilized. She gave birth to a son who is slightly affected. Her father had similar EMG and endplate abnormalities, but no symptoms of muscle weakness.

General remarks

Three arguments favor a diagnosis of the slow channel syndrome in this patient: the clinical syndrome with facial weakness and slowly progressive limb girdle type of weakness but no atrophy, the decrement and the double response on repetitive nerve stimulation, and the absence of AChR antibodies. The slow channel syndrome is a form of AD congenital myasthenia gravis caused by mutations in the AChR genes for one of the four subunits that form the adult receptor. The abnormal protein causes the receptor ion channel to stay open too long after stimulation with acetylcholine. This pathological gain in function causes

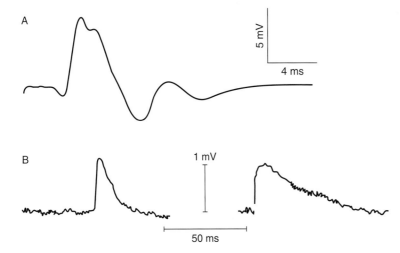

A

5 mV

4 ms

B

1 mV

50 ms

Figure 37.1. Repetitive CMAP in the abductor digiti minimi muscle evoked by a single stimulus to the ulnar nerve at the wrist (A). (B) Miniature endplate potentials in a biopsied intercostal muscle form a control subject (left) and a patient with the slow channel syndrome (right), which show an increase of the rise time and the decay time of this potential in the patient. These findings confirm that the AChR-ion channel stays open for too long. (From Oosterhuis HJGJ, Newsom-Davis J, Wokke JHJ, et al. The slow channel syndrome. Two new cases. *Brain* 1987; **110**: 1061–1079, with permission.)

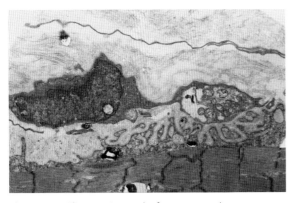

Figure 37.2. Electronmicrograph of a neuromuscular junction showing severe destruction of postsynaptic junctional folds at the extreme left. This is caused by calcium overload. The overlying presynaptic nerve terminal on the right will induce a new synaptic region nearby. The underlying muscle area shows loss of cross-striation, that is also caused by increased calcium influx. (x7000)

Table 37.1. How to proceed if congenital myasthenia gravis is suspected

- Clinical characteristics are exercise-induced muscle weakness, usually from childhood. Most patients have ptosis and delayed motor milestones
- EMG: search for decremental response
- Decrement, but no increment: analyze anti-AChR antibodies
- If negative: analyze anti-MuSK antibodies
- If negative, consider congenital myasthenia gravis
- EMG: search for a double response of the CMAP. A double response occurs in the slow channel syndrome and in AR endplate acetylcholinesterase deficiency, but not in other congenital myasthenic syndromes
- DNA analysis

myasthenic features. A second phenomenon is a calcium overload at the endplate, leading to destruction of the junctional folds and the subendplate muscle area.

Heredity of the slow channel syndrome is AD. Onset may be in later life and progression slow. Initially, cervical muscles and wrist and finger extensor muscles are selectively involved. Respiration may become insufficient, especially during respiratory tract infections or general anesthesia. Open-channel blockers of the AChR channel, such as quinidine sulphate, may be effective.

Other congenital myasthenic syndromes have AR inheritance and onset in infancy or childhood (Table 37.1). In the Netherlands, these include

patients with mutations in the rapsyn gene, the CHRNE gene – a gene encoding the epsilon subunits of the AChR, causing AChR deficiency, and mutations in the rapsyn gene.

Suggested reading

Beeson D. Congenital myasthenic syndromes. *Adv Clin Neurosci Rehabil* 2005; **4**: 12–13.

Burke G, Cossins J, Maxwell S, et al. Rapsyn mutations in hereditary myasthenia. *Neurology* 2003; **61**: 826–828.

Engel AG. Current status of the congenital myasthenic syndromes. *Neuromusc Disord* 2012; **22**: 99–111.

Engel AG, Ohno K, Sine SM. Sleuthing molecular targets for neurological disease at the neuromuscular junction. *Nat Rev Neurosci* 2003; **4**: 339–352.

Faber CG, Molenaar PC, Vles JSH, et al. AChR deficiency due epsilon-subunit mutations: two common mutations in the Netherlands. *J Neurol* 2009; **256**: 1719–1723.

Oosterhuis HJGJ, Newsom-Davis J, Wokke JHJ, et al. The slow channel syndrome. Two new cases. *Brain* 1987; **110**: 1061–1079.

CASE 38 Becker muscular dystrophy: two brothers who had difficulty climbing stairs

Clinical history

A 23-year-old electrotechnician gradually noticed difficulty running and climbing stairs. In retrospect, he had developed a hollow back at the age of 10 years, and when running, he had had difficulty keeping up with his peers.

Examination

There was hypertrophy of the proximal muscles of the upper and lower limbs, and of his calves (Figure 38.1). There was a positive Gowers' sign and a bilateral positive Trendelenburg sign (Video 17).

Ancillary investigations

Serum CK activity was elevated (15 × ULN). EMG, which was carried out by the referring neurologist,

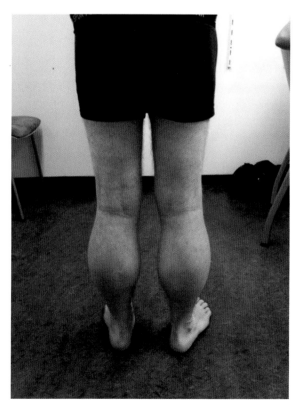

Figure 38.1. Hypertrophy of the calf muscles in a patient with Becker muscular dystrophy.

showed small motor unit action potentials. A CT scan of the muscular system demonstrated widespread abnormalities of muscles of the legs (Figure 38.2). A skeletal muscle biopsy showed dystrophic changes. Reduced dystrophin was observed on a Western blot (Figure 38.3). Mutation analysis of the dystrophin gene revealed a deletion of exons 45–47.

Diagnostic considerations

The limb girdle distribution of muscle weakness associated with a moderately elevated CK and a dystrophic muscle biopsy led to a clinical diagnosis of LGMD. A flowchart was used as a diagnostic guide (Figure 38.4). A diagnosis of Becker muscular dystrophy (BMD) was reached.

Follow-up

The patient was referred to the cardiology department where he was found to have a dilatation of the left ventricle with reduced function. He was prescribed an ACE-inhibitor and will be monitored annually.

After the patient was diagnosed, his brother was referred at the age of 20 years. He had been a keen baseball player until two years before, although he experienced muscle cramps on exertion and he was not as fast as his peers while running. On examination, he was found to have a limb girdle syndrome with additional winging of the scapulae, increased lumbar lordosis, and atrophy and slight weakness of the pectoralis major muscles. He also had atrophy of the upper leg muscles, hypertrophic calf muscles, and mild weakness of the foot extensor muscles. He had no cardiological abnormalities.

General remarks

BMD is caused by in-frame mutations in the dystrophin gene, which lead to reduced or otherwise altered dystrophin protein expression. The incidence of BMD is one-third of that of Duchenne muscular dystrophy (DMD: 1 in 2500–3500 live male births). The clinical picture of BMD is characterized by later age at onset and slower rate of progression compared to DMD. However, the spectrum of BMD encompasses a variety

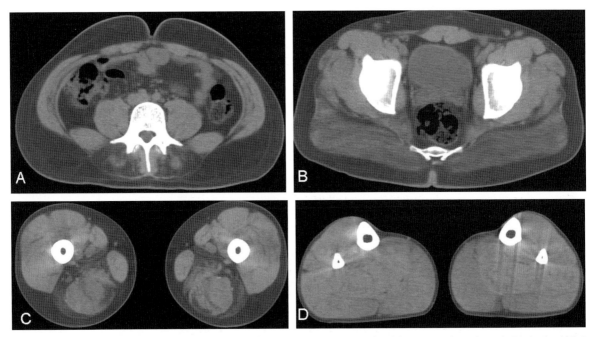

Figure 38.2. CT scan of a patient with Becker muscular dystrophy shows replacement by fat of the paraspinal muscles at the lumbar level (A). At the pelvic girdle level, there is lower attenuation of the gluteus maximus muscles (B), and at the thigh level of the adductor magnus, semimembranosus, and long head of the biceps femoris muscles, with compensatory hypertrophy of the gracilis muscles (C). The gastrocnemius muscles are hypertrophic (D).

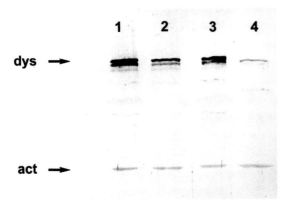

Figure 38.3. Lanes from a Western blot of skeletal muscle extract from three control subjects with normal dystrophin (dys, 1–3) and a patient with Becker muscular dystrophy showing reduced dystrophin (4). Actin (act) is present in equal amounts.

of phenotypes. These include an intermediate form between BMD and DMD ("outliers"), and a quadriceps-only form ("quadriceps myopathy"). Third, a very mild form exists in which BMD may manifest with myalgias and muscle cramps, exercise intolerance, and myoglobinuria, or even an asymptomatic slight elevation in the serum CK activity.

In most cases of BMD, the first symptoms are noticed between the sixth and eighteenth year of life with a mean age at onset of 11.1 years. The age at which ambulation is lost varies from 10 to 78 years (mean age is in the fourth decade).

Progressive dilated cardiomyopathy evolves in the same manner as DMD cardiomyopathy (Table 38.1). In BMD, the severity of cardiac disease does not correlate with that of skeletal muscle weakness. A severely dilated cardiomyopathy can occur in patients with BMD with relatively preserved skeletal muscle function.

Patients with BMD should undergo cardiac evaluation (electrocardiography and echocardiography) at diagnosis. They should be screened for the development of cardiomyopathy at least every five years, but preferably every two years. If progressive abnormalities are found, more regular monitoring is desirable together with treatment with ACE inhibitors and, if indicated, beta blockers. Cardiac transplantation may be a viable treatment option in this group of patients. Steroids that have some effect on disease progression of DMD are not effective in BMD.

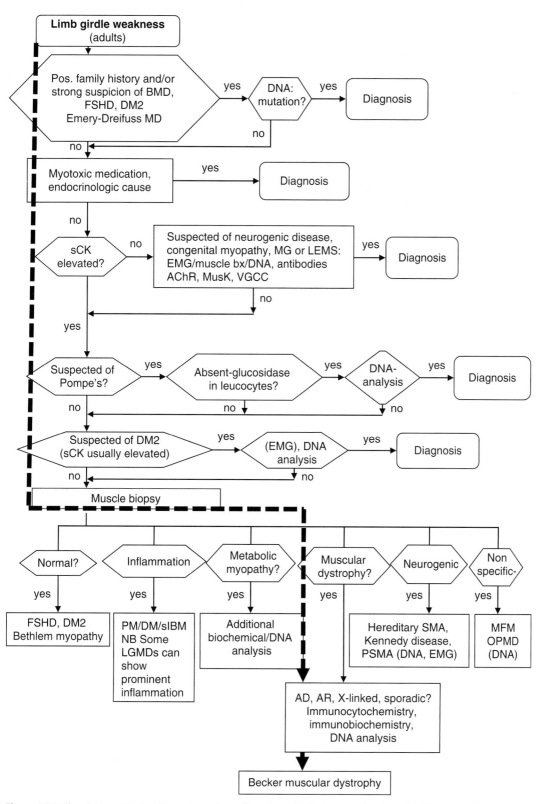

Figure 38.4. Flowchart used in the diagnostic work-up of a patient with Becker muscular dystrophy. The patient described presented with a limb girdle pattern of muscle weakness, had no positive family history for neuromuscular diseases, and had increased CK activity. DM type 1 was not suspected. The muscle biopsy showed a dystrophic pattern of abnormalities. Western blotting revealed a reduction in dystrophin. Subsequent DNA analysis confirmed the diagnosis.

Table 38.1. Cardiological abnormalities in neuromuscular disorders

Disease	Cardiac abnormalities	Case
Dystrophinopathies	Dilated cardiomyopathy	38 Female carriers may present with features of dilated cardiomyopathy
Caveolinopathy, including LGMD1C	Atrioventricular conduction defects, long QT-syndrome, dilated and hypertrophic cardiomyopathy	39 At present only rare cases described. Can be underestimation
Sarcoglycanopathies (LGMD2C-2F)	Dilated cardiomyopathy	Not discussed in this book as onset is during childhood in most cases
fukutin-related proteinopathy (LGMD2I)	Dilated cardiomyopathy	41
X-linked Emery–Dreifuss muscular dystrophy	Cardiac conduction abnormalities; atrial paralysis is pathognomonic	42 Female carriers may have conduction defects as well
AD Emery–Dreifuss muscular dystrophy 1 and 2/LGMD1B	Ventricular dysrhythmias, conduction defects, dilated or hypertrophic cardiomyopathy	42
Myofibrillar myopathies; e.g., desminopathy	Dilated cardiomyopathy	47
Danon disease	Males: hypertrophic cardiomyopathy Female carriers: dilated cardiomyopathy	X-linked lysosomal disorder with hypertrophic cardiomyopathy, myopathy and cognitive dysfunction/mental retardation caused by mutations in the lysosomal-associated membrane protein-2 (LAMP2) gene
Myotonic dystrophy type 1	Conduction defects and dysrhythmias Dilated cardiomyopathy during the course of the disease	50
Myotonic dystrophy type 2	Conduction defects and dysrhythmias Dilated cardiomyopathy during the course of the disease	51
Mitochondrial cytopathy	Hypertrophic cardiomyopathy, dilated cardiomyopathy, Wolff–Parkinson–White syndrome, other conduction abnormalities, dysrhythmias	55
Amyloidosis	Hypertrophic cardiomyopathy	Major cause of death in patients with familial amyloid polyneuropathy, usually with mutations in the transthyretrin gene (TTR). Also features of a length-dependent sensory, motor and autonomic neuropathy (pain, orthostasis) and liver failure caused by amyloid deposits
Guillain–Barré syndrome	Arrhythmias in acute and stable phase	14
Lyme radiculoneuritis	Grade 1 to 3 (complete) atrioventricular block, pericarditis and myocarditis can occur	27; generally good prognosis with treatment

LGMD: (see Table 41.1).

As more patients with neuromuscular diseases or neuromuscular manifestations of systemic disease are being recognized and results of long-term follow-up studies of these patients will become available in the future, this overview may have to be expanded.

Suggested reading

Hermans MC, Pinto YM, Merkies IS, et al. Hereditary muscular dystrophies and the heart. *Neuromuscul Disord* 2010; **20**: 479–492.

www.musclegenetable.fr

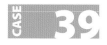

Caveolinopathy, including limb girdle muscular dystrophy type 1C: a janitor with muscle pains and cramps

Clinical history

A 47-year-old janitor had experienced exercise-induced muscle cramps from the age of 22 years. In his early forties, the cramps, myalgia, and stiffness were attributed to previously diagnosed hypothyroidism. Although progressive, he could continue to work. There were no family members with similar complaints.

Examination

He had generalized muscle hypertrophy, notably of the calves, but no weakness. Tapping or brief application of pressure to the upper arm or upper leg muscles produced short-lasting muscle contractions.

Ancillary investigations

Serum CK activity was twice the ULN. A muscle biopsy showed some atrophic fibers and reduced caveolin-3 expression in a Western blot analysis, but was otherwise normal. DNA analysis revealed a mutation in exon 1 of the gene for caveolin-3; c.142C>G;p. Pro48Ala.

Diagnostic considerations

A neurological examination in a patient presenting with myalgia and hyper-CK-emia is not complete without percussion of the muscles as this can easily (albeit in a very limited number of patients) lead to a correct diagnosis.

General remarks

Caveolin-3 is a membrane protein that is probably engaged in the formation of caveolae, small membrane invaginations that play a role in membrane transport and signal transduction. Reduced caveolin can be demonstrated in a muscle biopsy specimen (Figure 39.1). Mutations are usually AD transmitted. They may cause different phenotypes (Table 39.1).

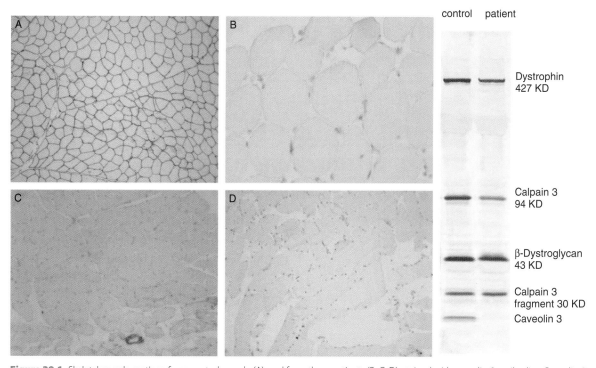

Figure 39.1. Skeletal muscle sections from control muscle (A), and from three patients (B, C, D), stained with caveolin-3 antibodies. Caveolin-3 expression was either severely reduced (B) or completely lost (C, D). Magnification x200 for (B) and x100 for (A, C, D). No caveolin-3 band was detectable on the Western blot of patient B. The bands for the other proteins were normal compared to the control. (From Aboumousa A, Hoogendijk J, Charlton R, et al. Caveolinopathy–new mutations and additional symptoms. *Neuromusc Disord* 2008; **18**: 572–578, with permission.)

Table 39.1. Phenotypes of caveolinopathy, caveolin-3 deficiency

- Myalgia
- Asymptomatic hyper-CK-emia
- LGMD1C
- Distal myopathy
- Rippling muscle disease with signs of hyperirritability such as rippling muscle movements, mounding, and percussion-induced rapid contractions

These phenotypes can appear on their own or in combination. There may be intrafamilial variation. Rippling muscle disease also exists as an acquired autoimmune disease (Case 18).

Many patients with a caveolinopathy present with myalgia and elevated CK levels without weakness. The neurological examination in a patient presenting with myalgia and hyper-CK-emia is not complete without percussion of the muscles, as this can lead to a "spot"-diagnosis, albeit in a very limited number of patients.

In these cases without apparent muscle weakness, a skeletal muscle biopsy may be normal or show aspecific myopathic features and even normal caveolin expression. On the other hand, secondary loss of caveolin-3 expression can be seen in other muscular dystrophies such as dysferlinopathy. Mutation analysis, therefore, is an important diagnostic tool.

Muscle rippling can also be the presenting symptom. Usually patients volunteer to show how they can evoke rippling and mounding by applying pressure to a muscle (Video 18). Percussion-induced rapid muscle contractions can easily be elicited by excercise, tapping, or stretching.

In children, the presenting symptom may be walking on tiptoe, but this is not usually accompanied by distal muscle weakness. In the limb girdle phenotype of LGMD1C, weakness is symmetric and affects shoulder girdle and hip girdle muscles, and sometimes interosseal and thumb muscles. Weakness is mild or moderate and does occur irrespective of disease duration in about half the patients. There is usually muscle hypertrophy, especially of the calves. Facial and bulbar weakness, scapular winging, respiratory insufficiency, and cranial involvement are not signs of caveolinopathy.

Cardiac abnormalities have been observed in patients with caveolinopathy (Table 38.1).

Suggested reading

Aboumousa A, Hoogendijk J, Charlton R, et al. Caveolinopathy – new mutations and additional symptoms. *Neuromuscul Disord* 2008; **18**: 572–578.

Gazzerro E, Sotgia F, Bruno C, Lisanti MP, Minetti C. Caveolinopathies: from the biology of caveolin-3 to human diseases. *Eur J Hum Genet* 2010; **18**: 137–145. [Erratum in: *Eur J Hum Genet* 2009; 17: 1692.]

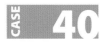

CASE 40 — Limb girdle muscular dystrophy type 2A, calpainopathy: an excellent soccer player who became severely handicapped over a period of 15 years

Clinical history

In his late twenties, this 30-year-old man reported difficulties lifting his arms and running, which progressed over subsequent years. During his teens he had been a very good soccer player.

Examination

There was bilateral symmetric scapular winging (Figure 40.1), symmetric wasting and weakness of elbow flexion, weakness of hip flexion and hip adduction, and bilateral calf hypertrophy. He had a pronounced lumbar lordosis and a waddling gait (Video 19). Contractures were not found. Respiratory and cardiac functions were normal.

Ancillary investigations

Serum CK activity was 40 × ULN. A CT scan showed fatty degeneration, especially of muscles that fixate the shoulder blade, elbow flexors, back extensors, hip adductors, and triceps surae muscles (Figure 40.2).

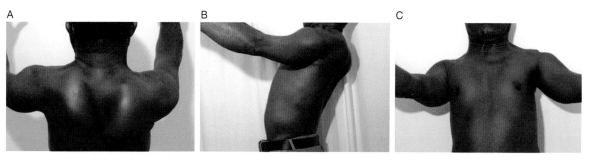

Figure 40.1. Bilateral symmetric scapular winging (A, B) and atrophy of muscles of upper arms (C).

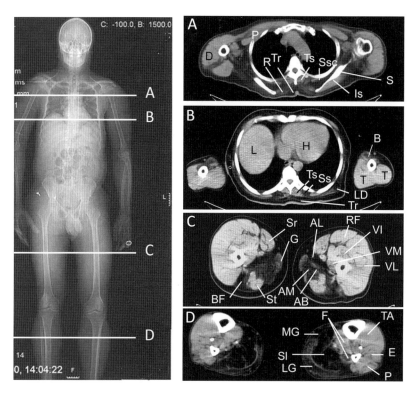

Figure 40.2. (see Figure 45.2, for comparison) CT shows replacement of various muscles by fat. At the shoulder girdle level (A, B): subscapular (Ssc), infraspinatus (Is), rhomboid (R), trapezius (Tr), latissimus dorsi (LD), sacrospinal (Ss), and biceps brachii (B) muscle. At the upper and lower leg level (C, D), biceps femoris (BF), adductor magnus (AM), adductor longus (AL), adductor brevis (AB), lateral head of gastrocnemius (LG); medial head of gastrocnemius (MG) and soleus muscle (Sl). S, scapula; L, liver; H, heart. The following muscles are relatively preserved: deltoid muscle (D), pectoral muscles (P), transversospinalis (Ts); triceps brachii (T); lateral vastus (VL); medial vastus (VM); intermedius vastus (VI); rectus femoris (RF); gracilis (G); sartorius (Sr); semitendinosus (St); anterior tibial (TA); peroneal muscles (P), toe flexors (F), and toe extensors (E).

Analysis of the CAPN3 gene revealed one mutation in exon 4: c.551C>T, p.Thr184Met and one as yet unclassified variant in exon 24.

Diagnostic considerations

This patient had onset of symptoms in early adulthood, symmetric scapular winging, weakness predominantly of elbow flexion more than extension and of hip adduction more than abduction, normal respiratory function, and very high CK. This combination of findings is highly suggestive of limb girdle muscular dystrophy (LGMD) type 2A.

Follow-up

Fifteen years after presentation, there was total loss of elbow flexion that – together with the loss of scapular fixation – made it almost impossible for him to use his arms. With great effort, he could walk for a few minutes. Cycling was impossible because of the tendency to fall when getting off the bike. Respiratory function, as measured by means of VC, was decreased (78% of expected).

General remarks

LGMD type 2A is caused by mutations in the calpain 3 (CAPN3) gene. It is a relatively common muscular

121

Table 40.1. Common clinical hallmarks of limb girdle muscular dystrophy type 2A, calpainopathy

- Onset in late childhood or adolescence
- Symmetric scapular winging with atrophy of scapular, pelvis, and trunk muscles
- Contractures may be found: ankle dorsiflexion, finger flexion, elbow flexion, and wrist flexion
- Specific pattern of muscle involvement with predominant weakness of elbow flexors, hip adductors, flexors, and extensors, and knee flexors
- Relative preservation of elbow extension, hip abduction, and knee extension, and of distal muscles
- Normal respiratory function
- (Very) high CK activity

dystrophy. Inheritance is AR. Typically, patients report completely normal muscle function prior to the first symptoms of upper leg weakness, which usually presents in their teens (Table 40.1). As a consequence, the gait is waddling and sometimes tiptoeing, with increased lumbar lordosis. Respiratory and cardiac functions remain normal. Atrophy of selected muscles may occur (Video 20). Furthermore, CK activity is strongly increased. On average, ambulation is lost two decades after onset of the symptoms. Intrafamilial variability has been observed with respect to age of onset and clinical course. Rehabilitation therapy should be offered to all patients.

Identification of calpain 3 protein abnormalities by Western blot analysis is neither very specific nor very sensitive. Currently, DNA analysis is not always conclusive, as in a minority of patients with a typical LGMD2A phenotype, only one mutation in the CAPN3 gene can be detected.

Suggested reading

Bushby KM. Diagnosis and management of the limb girdle muscular dystrophies. *Pract Neurol* 2009; **9**: 314–323.

Groen EJ, Charlton R, Barresi R, et al. Analysis of the UK diagnostic strategy for limb girdle muscular dystrophy 2A. *Brain* 2007; **130**: 3237–3249.

Saenz A, Leturcq F, Cobo AM, et al. LGMD2A: genotype-phenotype correlations based on a large mutational survey on the calpain 3 gene. *Brain* 2005; **128**: 732–742.

Schessl J, Walter MC, Schreiber G, et al. Phenotypic variability in siblings with calpainopathy (LGMD2A). *Acta Myol* 2008; **27**: 54–58.

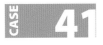

CASE 41

Limb girdle muscular dystrophy type 2I, fukutin-related protein deficiency: An anesthesiology nurse with backache

Clinical history

A 41-year-old man was referred because of persistent backache. When questioned he recalled that he had had firm calves since childhood. Once, after strenuous exercise, he had experienced coffee coloured urine,

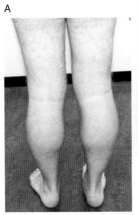
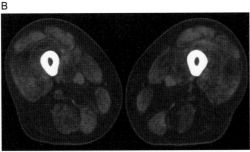

Figure 41.1. Hypertrophy of the calves (A). CT scan shows areas of lower attenuation in all upper leg muscles, suggesting wasting and fatty replacement (B).

strongly suggestive of myoglobinuria. At the time, he did not consult his GP.

Examination

He had hypertrophic calves and weakness of the hip flexors (Figure 41.1). Gowers' sign was positive. Otherwise, the neurological examination was normal.

Ancillary investigations

Serum CK activity was 15 × ULN. A CT scan of the muscular system showed diffuse changes of the pelvic girdle and upper leg muscles, suggesting wasting and fatty replacement (Figure 41.1). A skeletal muscle biopsy showed moderate variation in the muscle fibers and scattered necrotic and regenerating fibers. Dystrophin

Table 41.1. Classifications of the limb girdle muscular dystrophies

Type 1 autosomal dominant	Gene	Protein	Onset
LGMD1A	TTID	Myotilin	Variable
LGMD1B	LMNA	Lamin A/C	Variable
LGMD1C	CAV3	Caveolin 3	Variable
LGMD1D	Unknown		Adulthood
LGMD1E	Unknown		2nd decade and later
LGMD1F	Unknown		Variable
LGMD1G	Unknown		Adulthood
LGMD1H	Unknown		Variable
Type 2 autosomal recessive	**Gene**	**Protein**	**Onset**
LGMD2A	CAPN3	Calpain 3	Variable
LGMD2B	DYSF	Dysferlin	Adolescence and early adulthood
LGMD2C	SGCG	γ-Sarcoglycan	Early childhood
LGMD2D	SGCA	α-Sarcoglycan	Early childhood
LGMD2E	SGCB	β-Sarcoglycan	Early childhood
LGMD2F	SGCD	δ-Sarcoglycan	Early childhood
LGMD2G	TCAP	Telethonin	2nd decade
LGMD2H	TRIM 32	Tripartite motif containing 32	Adulthood
LGMD2I	FKRP	Fukutin-related protein	Variable
LGMD2J	TTN	Titin	(Early) adulthood
LGMD2K	POMT1	Protein-O-mannosyltransferase 1	Childhood
LGMD2L	ANO5	Anoctamin 5	2nd decade–adulthood
LGMD2M	FKTN	Fukutin	Early childhood
LGMD2N	POMT2	Protein-O-mannosyltransferase 2	Early childhood
LGMD2O	POMGnT1	Protein O-linked mannose beta1, 2-N-Acetylglucosaminyltransferase	Early childhood
LGMD2P	DAG1	Dystroglycan	Early childhood
LGMD2Q	PLEC1	Plectin	Early childhood

Adapted from Nigro V, Aurino S, Piluso G. Limb girdle muscular dystrophies: update on genetic diagnosis and therapeutic approaches. *Curr Opin Neurol* 2011; **24**: 429–436.
For LGMD1D-H, no genes have yet been identified.
As more patients with LGMD are being recognized, the variation of phenotypes will increase.
In this book, we have focused upon patients who experienced first manifestations during late adolescence or in adulthood. Diseases that manifest in children have been included for completeness. (See www.musclegenetable.fr, www.neuromuscular.wustl.edu)

and other membrane markers were present in normal amounts, but alpha-dystroglycan was reduced. Mutation analysis of the fukutin-related protein (FRKP)-gene was performed revealing a homozygous missense mutation, which was consistent with a diagnosis of LGMD type 2I.

Diagnostic considerations

The presence of limb girdle distribution of muscle weakness associated with moderately elevated CK activity and a dystrophic muscle biopsy led to a differential diagnosis of LGMD (Table 41.1). LGMD2I was diagnosed using a protocol with skeletal muscle protein and mutation analysis.

Follow-up

The patient had no cardiac involvement at presentation, but during follow-up after two years he was found to have developed left ventricular dysfunction He died suddenly while waiting for implantation of an implantable cardioverter defibrillator.

General remarks

The prevalence of LGMD2I varies between populations. In the Netherlands, 8% of all LGMD families have LGMD2I, whereas it is one of the most prevalent LGMDs in the United Kingdom and Denmark. LGMD2I, caused by mutations in the fukutin-related protein (FKRP) gene, is an autosomal recessive disorder. The FKRP-gene is a homolog of the fukutin gene encoding for the fukutin-related protein. FKRP is a putative glycosyltransferase, the precise function of which is uncertain. It has been localized in the Golgi apparatus and is involved in the glycosylation processing of alpha-dystroglycan, an indispensable molecule for binding laminin alpha 2. FKRP is ubiquitously expressed. Mutations in the FKRP gene located on chromosome 19q13 can give rise to a congenital muscular dystrophy (MDC1C), a Walker–Warburg syndrome (congenital muscular dystrophy, hydrocephalus, agyria, and retinal dysplasia) and a relatively mild form of LGMD (LGMD2I).

The disease severity of LGMD2I is variable. A late onset is associated with a mild course as far as muscle weakness is concerned. Calf hypertrophy is found in a majority of the cases which can cause confusion with Becker muscular dystrophy. The same holds true for exertional pain and muscle cramps. Myoglobinuria is observed in 25% of the cases.

Left ventricular hypokinesis, dilated cardiomyopathy, and heart failure have been reported in about one-third of LGMD2I patients, regardless of the gene mutation and the severity of the muscular disease, suggesting that all patients should be referred for cardiac evaluation (see Table 38.1). All patients with LGDM2I should be evaluated for cardiac involvement (electrocardiography and echocardiography) at diagnosis. Subsequent two-year screening would seem advisable.

Suggested reading

Nigro V, Aurino S, Piluso G. Limb girdle muscular dystrophies: update on genetic diagnosis and therapeutic approaches. *Curr Opin Neurol* 2011; **24**: 429–436.

Sveen ML, Schwartz M, Vissing J. High prevalence and phenotype–genotype correlations of limb girdle muscular dystrophy type 2I in Denmark. *Ann Neurol* 2006; **59**: 808–815.

Van der Kooi AJ, Frankhuizen WS, Barth PG, et al. Limb-girdle muscular dystrophy in the Netherlands: gene defect identified in half the families. *Neurology* 2007; **68**: 2125–2128.

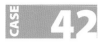

Emery–Dreifuss muscular dystrophy: two brothers with contractures

Clinical history

The youngest of five children of Turkish origin noticed at the age of five years that he was not able to fully extend his arms. Furthermore, his Achilles tendons were taut. His previous history was unremarkable. An older brother had similar symptoms. He had no cardiac symptoms.

Examination

At the age of 24 years, he was found to have a rigid spine and neck (Figure 42.1), contractures at the elbows and shortening of the Achilles tendons, scoliosis and increased lumbar lordosis.

There was atrophy of the muscles of the lower arms and legs, and he had scapulae alatae. Mild weakness of the triceps brachii and iliopsoas muscles was observed. He had generalized areflexia.

Ancillary investigations

Cardiological examination showed a first degree AV-block. Serum CK activity was 715 IU/L (normal, <171 IU/L).

Diagnostic considerations

Contractures and muscle weakness can be found in a number of neuromuscular conditions (Table 42.1). However, scapuloperoneal muscle weakness, contractures, and cardiac involvement are consistent with X-linked recessive or AD Emery–Dreifuss muscular dystrophy. DNA analysis revealed a missense mutation (c.3G>A) in the STA-gene (emerin gene) on chromosome Xq28.

General remarks

In the 1960s, this novel variant of X-linked muscular dystrophy was described and characterized by:

A
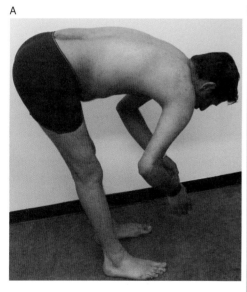

B
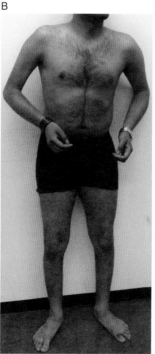

Figure 42.1. Rigid spine (A), and elbow contractures and atrophy of the muscles of the lower arms and legs (B).

Table 42.1. Contractures and muscle weakness in neuromuscular disorders

Muscular dystrophies

X-linked recessive Emery–Dreifuss muscular dystrophy

AD and AR Emery–Dreifuss muscular dystrophy

Other muscular dystrophies; e.g., LGMD2A (calpain 3 gene)

Bethlem myopathy

Dermatomyositis

Congenital myopathy

Rigid-spine syndromes

- Selenoprotein-related myopathy (SEPN1-gene): onset from birth to the second decade of life
- Four-and-a-half LIM domain protein 1 (FHL1)-related myopathies: onset can be in adulthood

Some forms of nemaline myopathy (arthrogryposis: diagnosed before or after birth, or in infancy)

Congenital muscular dystrophies

- *Fukuyama congenital muscular dystrophy*
- *Merosin-deficient congenital muscular dystrophy*
- *Ullrich congenital muscular dystrophy*

Neonatal myasthenia gravis–these features are transient except for congenital arthrogryposis caused by maternal antibodies versus fetal AChRs, usually in untreated mothers with myasthenia gravis

Congenital AR spinal muscular atrophy (arthrogryposis of mainly the lower leg, usually not progressive), also known as SMA-LED

The diseases that are presented in italics may manifest with contractures in neonates and children.

- Early contractures – often preceding muscle weakness – of the Achilles tendons, elbows, and posterior cervical muscles (rigid neck) but no torticollis. Limitation of forward flexion of the thoracic and lumbar spine (rigid spine) occurs later.
- Slowly progressive muscle weakness with a humeroperoneal or limb girdle distribution, rarely leading to wheelchair dependency.
- Dilated cardiomyopathy and atrioventricular conduction defects are almost invariably present and usually appear after the second decade of life, irrespective of contractures or muscle weakness (Table 38.1). Even complete heart block can occur. Occasional sudden death without preceding cardiac symptoms warrants preventive pacemaker

implantation. This may also occur in asymptomatic female carriers.

- There is considerable inter- and intrafamilial variation.
- Ancillary investigations are usually noncontributory. Serum CK is slightly to moderately elevated (up to 20 × ULN). The muscle biopsy shows a dystrophic picture with absent emerin staining. The diagnosis is established by DNA analysis. X-linked Emery–Dreifuss muscular dystrophy is caused by mutations in the EMD gene, encoding a protein named emerin. The differential diagnosis (Table 42.1) includes AD Emery–Dreifuss muscular dystrophy, which has the same clinical picture but is caused by LMNA mutations on chromosome 1, encoding lamins A and C (LGMD type 1B). Cardiac evaluation is obligatory in X-linked and AD Emery–Dreifuss muscular dystrophy (see Table 38.1). One should also consider the Emery–Dreifuss phenotype caused by mutations in the following genes: FHL1 (four-and-a-half-LIM) gene, SYNE-1 (synaptic nuclear envelope protein 1 or Nesprin), SYNE-2, TMEM43 (encoding for LUMA), and Bethlem myopathy caused by mutations in one of the three collagen VI genes. Cardiac manifestations are absent in Bethlem myopathy.
- All but FHL1 are nuclear envelope proteins. Emerin is an inner nuclear membrane protein, essential for the structural integrity of the nucleus. Lamins are proteins that form nuclear laminae and anchor inner nuclear membrane proteins. They thus help to provide a mechanical, resistant meshwork. These and other proteins function as a scaffold for the cytoskeleton.
- Other disorders with contractures can be found in the table. Congenital muscular dystrophies and congenital AR SMA manifest directly after birth. Decreased childhood movements and arthrogryposis are evidence of even earlier onset.

Suggested reading

Helbling-Leclerc A, Bonne G, Schwartz K. Emery–Dreifuss muscular dystrophy. *Eur J Hum Genet* 2002; **10**: 157–161.

Liang W-C, Mitsuhashi H, Keduka E, et al. TMEM43 mutations in Emery–Dreifuss muscular dystrophy-related myopathy. *Ann Neurol* 2011; **69**: 1005–1013.

Facioscapulohumeral dystrophy: a woman who had a problem walking and pain in one arm

Clinical history

In her early forties, a 51-year-old woman first noticed fatigue when walking. She attributed this to hollowing of her back and tendencies to push her tummy forward and allow it to protrude. Later on, she noticed difficulty and pain in lifting her right arm. She had never been able to whistle properly. Her parents and sisters did not have muscle complaints.

Examination

When attempting to pout the lips, there was a slight inability to contract the lower lip completely on one side (Figure 43.1). There was a scapula alata on the right side and possibly also on the left. She could not stand on her heels without sticking her buttocks out. When walking, there was lumbar hyperlordosis.

Ancillary investigations

Serum CK activity was slightly elevated (2 × ULN). DNA analysis showed a normal EcoRI/BlnI fragment as detected by the P13E-11 probe, but methylation-sensitive Southern blot analysis revealed a loss of D4Z4 methylation levels confirming the clinical diagnosis of facioscapulohumeral dystrophy (FSHD).

Diagnostic considerations

The phenotype was typical for FSHD. Many patients with FSHD present with unilateral shoulder and arm or shoulder pain, probably as result of chronic overuse. In 95% of patients with a typical FSHD phenotype, the diagnosis can be confirmed relatively easily by showing a deletion in the D4Z4-repeat on chromosome 4qter.

Follow-up

In the course of five years, walking became more difficult. She had to use a rollator for longer distances.

General remarks

FSHD is one of the most common hereditary myopathies. The estimated prevalence is approximately 10 per 100 000 of the general population. The disease is AD transmitted. A substantial proportion of cases are due to a de novo mutation. In 95% of cases (FSHD1), the disease is caused by a contraction of the macrosatellite repeat array D4Z4 in the subtelomeric region of chromosome 4q. Patients with FSHD have only 1–10 repeats whereas healthy individuals have 11–150 repeats. This deletion results in local chromatin relaxation and stable expression of the D4Z4-encoded DUX4 gene. DUX4 is a transcription gene that may target other genes. Activation of the DUX4 gene causes a deregulation cascade inhibiting myogenesis. In addition, FSHD occurs only in association with certain haplotypes that are associated with a polyadenylation signal distal of the last D4Z4 unit. Large deletions in the D424 repeat can be associated with earlier onset, more rapid progression, and more severe disease. DNA hypomethylation in D4Z4 repeats in the presence of the 4A161 haplotype also occurs in patients with a typical FSHD phenotype but lacking the D4Z4 deletion.

A
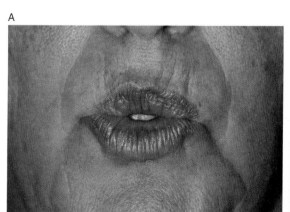

B
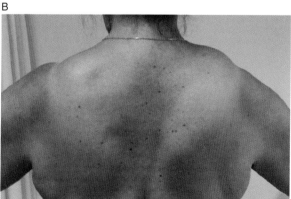

Figure 43.1. Slightly asymmetric and incomplete pouting of the lips (A) and asymmetric winging of the shoulder blades (B). Note the abnormal contour of the right shoulder.

The SMHCDI gene on chromosome 18 seems implicated in FSHD 2 patients. Patients without the D4Z4 deletion have FSHD2 with the identical clinical presentation to FSHD1.

Disease severity and age at onset vary widely, even within sibships, but the distribution and route of progression of weakness is fairly characteristic. Facial muscles, especially the orbicularis oris muscle, and scapular fixators are the first to become weak. Many patients recall that they have never been able to drink through a straw. Orbicularis oris weakness may be subtle and only apparent on the patient's attempt to whistle. Weakness is typically asymmetric, and asymmetric lip closure and winging scapulae allow a spot diagnosis, which can be confirmed relatively easily by DNA analysis in FSHD1.

Classic cases have problems with fixation of the shoulder to the trunk while lifting the arms (see Introduction, Figure 14). Usually the deltoid muscle is relatively spared, but its function is hampered by the loose scapula. Winging of the scapulae will become more evident when the patient presses the outstretched arms firmly against a hard surface (see Introduction, Figure 15). Progression of weakness subsequently involves upper arm muscles, foot dorsiflexors, abdominal wall and paraspinal muscles, and proximal leg muscles. Approximately 20% of patients become wheelchair bound. There is usually no cardiac involvement. Some severely affected patients suffer from respiratory insufficiency. Atypical phenotypes of FSHD have been recognized (Table 43.1). Severity of weakness may differ greatly between patients.

Management of patients with FSHD includes genetic counseling and rehabilitation care. Surgical

Table 43.1. Atypical phenotypes of facioscapulohumeral dystrophy

- Facial-sparing with scapular winging
- Limb girdle syndrome
- Axial myopathy with bent spine syndrome
- Distal myopathy with frequently asymmetric foot drop, rarely calf weakness
- Asymmetric arm weakness
- Exclusive involvement of the calves

scapular fixation has been reported to be successful, but no consensus exists.

Suggested reading

Cabianca DS, Gabellini D. The cell biology of disease: FSHD: copy number variations on the theme of muscular dystrophy. *J Cell Biol* 2010; **191**: 1049–1060.

De Greef JS, Lemmers RJ, Camaño P, et al. Clinical features of facioscapupulohumeral dystrophy 2. *Neurology* 2010; **75**: 1548–1554.

Lemmers RJ, Tawil R, Petek LM, et al. Digenic inheritance of an SMCHD1 mutation and an FSHD-permissive D4Z4 allele cause facioscapulohumeral muscular dystrophy type 2. *Nat Genet* 2012; **44**: 1370–374.

Richards M, Coppée F, Thomas N, Belayew A, Upadhyaya M. Facioscapulohumeral muscular dystrophy (FSHD): an enigma unravelled? *Hum Genet* 2012; **131**: 325–340.

Van der Maarel SM, Tawil R, Tapscott SJ. Facioscapulohumeral muscular dystrophy and DUX4: breaking the silence. *Trends Mol Med* 2011; **17**: 252–258.

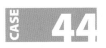

CASE 44 Miyoshi distal myopathy, dysferlin myopathy: a student with thinning of both calves

Clinical history

A 24-year-old student in technical engineering complained of instability of his feet since the age of 16 years. From the age of 19 years onward, he could no longer stand on tiptoe, and he experienced difficulties when playing basketball. At 20 years of age, his calves appeared to be thin. Gradually, he had some difficulty running, whereas he could climb the stairs and rise from a chair normally. He had no symptoms in his arms. The family history was negative.

Examination

He had normal posture and the musculature of his arms, trunk, and upper legs was well developed and of normal strength. There were no contractures nor scoliosis. Both calves, but also the anterior muscles of the lower legs, were thin (Figure 44.1). He had weakness of the gastrocnemius, soleus, flexor digitorum, and peroneal muscles, MRC grade 4–5. Sensation was normal. Achilles tendon reflexes were absent. He had difficulty tiptoeing. To compensate for the calf muscle weakness, he could walk only on his toes while bending his knees.

A B

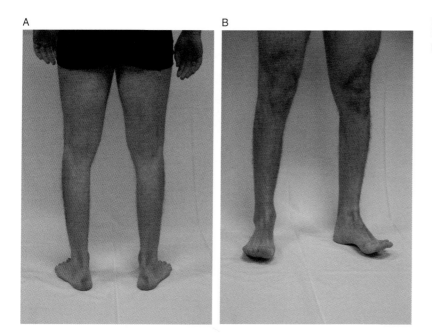

Figure 44.1. Atrophy of both calves (A), but also of the foot extensor muscles. The patient cannot stand on his heels (B).

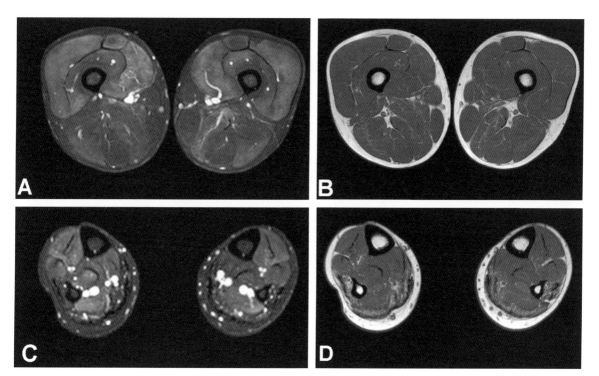

Figure 44.2. Transverse 1.5T MRI scans of the corresponding sections of the upper legs (A, T2-STIR; B, T1 weighted) and through the mid-calves (C, T2-STIR; D, T1 weighted).

Ancillary investigations

Serum CK activity was 15,820 IU/L (>90 × ULN). ECG was normal. MRI showed edema in unaffected muscles of both upper legs and replacement of the gastrocnemius muscles by fat (Figures 44.2 and 44.3). Next, two unclassified variants in exons 12 and 47 of the dysferlin gene were indentified. Both parents carried one of these

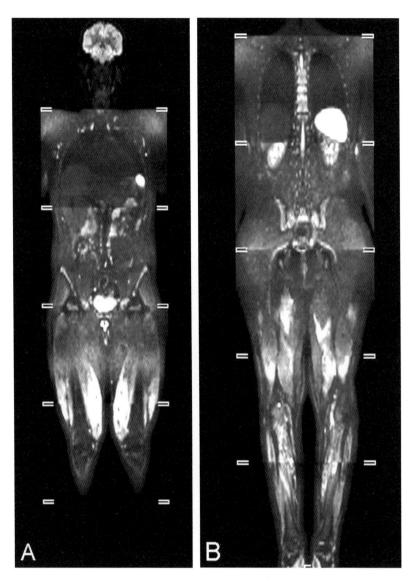

Figure 44.3. T2-STIR MRI coronal sections through anterior (A) and posterior (B) parts of legs. The presence of edema is evident in the quadriceps femoris and the posterior muscles.

variants. We hypothesized that a dysferlinopathy was likely and for confirmation took a skeletal muscle biopsy of the left vastus lateral muscle to analyze for dysferlin. Histopathological analysis of the biopsy showed dystrophic abnormalities (Figure 44.4). Immunohistochemical analysis revealed an absence of dysferlin. Western blotting showed an absence of dysferlin in the presence of normal dystrophin and calpain-3 (Figure 44.4).

Diagnostic considerations

The hallmarks of this case are gradual onset in adolescence, predominant atrophy and weakness of both calves, and a markedly elevated serum CK activity.

EMG can be omitted as CK elevation >10 × ULN excludes axonal neuropathy, distal SMA and a conus-cauda tumor. As this patient had two currently unclassified variants in both dysferlin genes, we analyzed dysferlin in a muscle biopsy.

Several hereditary myopathies are, at onset or during the course of the disease, characterized by predominant involvement of the posterior compartments of the leg (Table 44.1).

General remarks

The plasma membrane, sarcolemma, is an important part of the skeletal muscle fiber wall. It acts as a

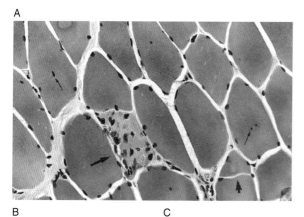

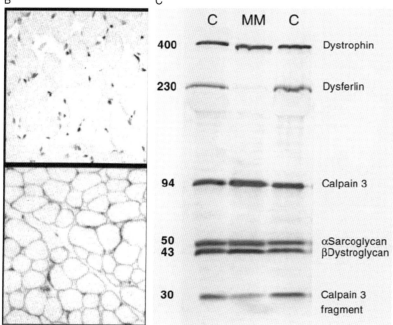

Figure 44.4. Skeletal muscle biopsy of the lateral vastus muscle of a patient with dysferlinopathy showing a necrotic muscle fibre (A, arrow), absent dysferlin staining (B, upper row; control biopsy with positive staining in lower row), and virtually absent dysferlin with Western blot (C, middle lane).

biological barrier between extracellular and intracellular environments and maintains cell integrity. Minor physiological disruptions occur frequently in active skeletal muscle cells. Active membrane repair mechanisms aimed at resealing these lesions, have been conserved in many types of mammalian cells. Dysferlin is involved in Ca^{2+}-dependent membrane repair. Calpains may also be required for efficient membrane repair. Deficiency of muscle-specific proteins, caveolin-3 and calpain-3, cause distinct muscular dystrophies (caveolinopathy can manifest as LGMD1C and distal myopathy, and calpainopathy is characterized as LGMD2A). Both proteins interact with dysferlin, but their exact role in muscle

membrane repair is unknown. Patients with dysferlinopathy have reduced levels of calpain-3, and patients with caveolinopathy have reduced or mislocalized dysferlin. Anoctamin 5 may also play a role in defective membrane repair.

Dysferlin is a 230 kDa protein and part of the ferlin-1-like proteins. The protein is not part of the dystrophin–glycoprotein complex that links the cytoskeleton to the surrounding basement membrane. Mutations in the dysferlin gene cause three clinically distinct phenotypes (Table 44.2).

The heart is not affected.

Recent MRI of leg muscles showed a huge overlap of abnormalities between patients with distal Miyoshi

all

Table 44.1. Hereditary myopathies with predominant involvement of the posterior muscles of the lower leg

Dysferlinopathy

- First described in Japan in 1977; ubiquitous Miyoshi myopathy
- Inheritance AR
- Onset in late adulthood
- Most patients wheelchair-bound after a few decades
- Early on in the disease, involvement of gluteus medius muscles (MRI)
- Biceps brachii muscle first muscle affected in the upper limb

Distal myopathy with mutations in the anoctamin 5 gene

- Inheritance AR
- LGMD2L or distal myopathy manifesting with calf muscle weakness: Miyoshi muscular dystrophy type 3 (MMD3)
- CK elevation manifold
- Onset usually decade later compared with Miyoshi myopathy
- More protracted disease course
- Asymmetry of muscle atrophy or weakness

Distal myopathy due to mutation in the myotilin gene

- Inheritance: AD.
- Weakness of anterior more than posterior lower leg muscles
- Onset between 50 and 60 years of age
- Some patients present with calf muscle weakness
- CK elevation mild (<4 x ULN)
- Rimmed and nonrimmed vacuoles and desmin–myotilin aggregates in muscle biopsy

Posterior lower leg muscle weakness manifests at onset or during the course of the disease.

Table 44.2. Phenotypes associated with mutations in the dysferlin gene

- Distal Miyoshi myopathy with early gastrocnemius muscle involvement
- Limb girdle muscular dystrophy type 2 B (LGMD2B) that is characterized by proximal muscle weakness at onset
- Rare: distal anterior compartment myopathy with weakness of the anterior tibial muscles
- Extremely rare: congenital muscular dystrophy, scapuloperoneal syndrome, isolated hyper-CK-emia

myopathy or LGMD2B phenotypes. In some families, both phenotypes are present. The cause of these variations in and between families is not known. Inheritance is AR. The genotype does not predict the phenotype or progression. The term, dysferlin myopathy, is probably more appropriate for all cases. Treatment is symptomatic with a prominent role for rehabilitation.

Suggested reading

Han R, Campbell KP. Dysferlin and muscle membrane repair. *Curr Opin Cell Biol* 2007; **19**: 409–416.

Hicks D, Sarkozy A, Muelas N, et al. A founder mutation in anoctamin 5 is a major cause of limb-girdle muscular dystrophy. *Brain* 2011; **134**: 171–182.

Paradas C, Llauger J, Diaz-Manera J et al. Redefining dysferlinopathy phenotypes based on clinical findings and muscle imaging studies. *Neurology* 2010; **75**: 316–323.

Udd B. Genetics and pathogenesis of distal muscular dystrophies. *Adv Exp Med Biol* 2009; **652**: 23–38.

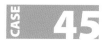
Distal myopathy with rimmed vacuoles, hereditary inclusion body myopathy: a young man with thin lower legs who could not walk on his heels

Clinical history

This 21-year-old man had complained for some years of diffuse pain and weakness of the legs. His sister was reported to have a severe disorder of the nerves or muscles. Their parents were believed not to be related. The family is of Turkish ancestry.

Examination

There was mild symmetric atrophy of the anterior tibial muscles and the medial gastrocnemius muscles and a hammer toe deformity. We found normal strength of both arms, but mild weakness in the hip adductor and gastrocnemius muscles (MRC 4–5), and moderate weakness of the foot dorsal flexors (MRC 4) and toe dorsal flexor muscles (MRC 3–4). Sensation was normal. Tendon reflexes could be elicited. Figure 45.1 shows the patient nine years after presentation.

Ancillary investigations

Serum CK was elevated (6 × ULN). Needle EMG showed positive sharp waves and fibrillation potentials and short-duration, low-voltaged muscle action potentials. MCNVs and SNCVs were normal. He declined a skeletal muscle biopsy as in his sister the biopsy of the lateral vastus muscle had shown only aspecific myopathic changes. Muscle imaging, by means of MRI nine years after initial presentation, to examine the level of involvement of various muscles, showed severe abnormalities (Figure 45.2). As he was diagnosed with a distal myopathy and his sister was reported to be severely affected, an AR hereditary distal myopathy was considered a likely explanation. The next step was DNA analysis of the UDP-GlcNAc 2-Epimerase/ManNAckinase gene (GNE) that showed a homozygous c.172C>T p.P58S mutation.

Diagnostic considerations

This patient presented with distal more than proximal weakness of both legs that had existed for many years. The complaints of pain could be attributed to chronic over-use. The muscle biopsy in his affected sister showed only aspecific abnormalities, but no rimmed vacuoles. The absence of diagnostic abnormalities can possibly be explained by the fact that the biopsy was taken from an

A

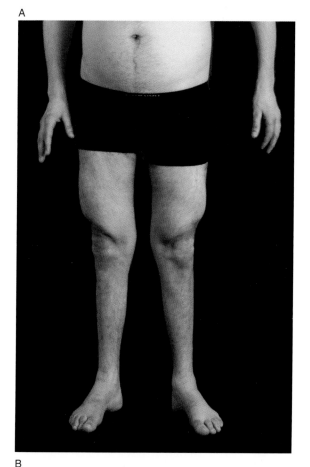

B

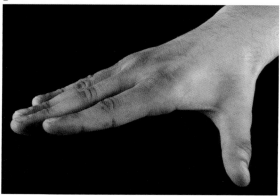

Figure 45.1. (A) Severe atrophy of the muscles of the lower legs with sparing of the quadriceps femoris muscles (compare with sporadic inclusion body myositis and CMT disease). He had severe atrophy of the first interosseus muscles (B).

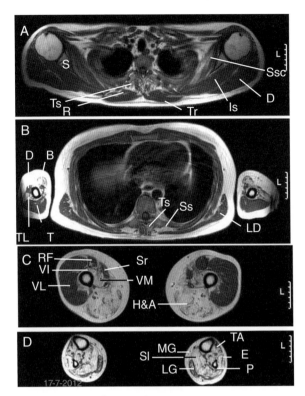

Figure 45.2. (see Figure 40.2, for comparison) Transverse T1-weighted sections at the level of the shoulders (A), proximal upper arm (B), proximal upper leg (C), and mid-lower leg (D), showing prominent symmetric atrophy and fatty degeneration of the biceps brachii muscle (B), the lateral head of the triceps brachii muscle (TL), the sacrospinal muscle (Ss), the complete medial and posterior compartment of the upper leg (with relative sparing of the sartorius muscle [Sr]), the medial vastus muscle (VM), the vastus intermedius muscle (VI), and all muscles of the lower leg. D, deltoid muscle; E, toe extensors (dorsal flexors); H&A, hamstring and adductor muscles; Is, infraspinatus muscle; LD, latissimus dorsi muscle; LG, lateral head of gastrocnemius muscle; MG, medial head of gastrocnemius muscle; P, peroneal muscles; R, rhomboid muscle; RF, rectus femoris muscle; S, scapula; Ssc, subscapular muscle; Sl, soleus muscle; T, triceps; TA, anterior tibial muscle; Tr, trapezius muscle; Ts, transversospinal muscle; VL, lateral vastus muscle.

asymptomatic muscle. Muscle imaging can be helpful in many myopathies to show specific patters of muscle involvement. In this patient, muscle imaging showed relative sparing of the quadriceps muscles, which prompted the investigation of the GNE gene.

Follow-up

Nine years after presentation he had difficulty climbing stairs and holding heavy objects. He tried ankle–foot ortheses because of foot drop, but this did not suit him. His VC was 108% of expected and there were no cardiac abnormalities. He had symmetric

Table 45.1. Myopathies with prominent distal involvement

- Distal myopathies: myopathies with predominant distal weakness (see Tables 44.1 and 45.2)
- Caveolinopathy
- Facioscapulohumeral dystrophy
- Oculopharyngeal distal myopathy
- Scapuloperoneal syndrome (desminopathy)
- Myotonic dystrophy type
- sIBM

Distal muscle weakness forms part of the clinical spectrum of telethoninopathy (LGMD2G).

weakness of biceps brachii and finger flexor muscles, MRC 4; iliopsoas and toe plantar flexor muscles, MRC 3; hamstring muscles, and ankle plantar flexor muscles MRC 2, hip adductor and all other distal leg muscles MRC 0.

General remarks

If a patient presents with distal weakness, the diagnostic process should start with differentiating between a distal myopathy and a disease of motor neurons or nerves. Unilateral or asymmetric weakness can be observed in acquired diseases, both neurogenic and myopathic. Neurogenic causes are segmental ALS, SMA, and MMN. Sporadic IBM is a myopathy with unilateral or asymmetric weakness. Symmetric presentation in general indicates hereditary disease, which can be neurogenic (e.g., distal SMA) or myopathic. In myopathies, distal weakness occasionally may be an early or prominent sign of a more generalized disease. Examples are DM type 1 and FSHD (Table 45.1). In true distal myopathies, distal weakness is present at the onset of the disease. During the course of the disease, weakness remains more distal than proximal. Some genes involved in a distal myopathy can also be causative in proximal myopathies (Table 45.2). Examples of these are the dysferlin (Case 44), desmin (Case 47), and myotilin genes.

Numerous different entities of distal myopathies are recognized currently and several of these can be diagnosed by molecular genetic analyses. The diagnostic process of hereditary distal myopathies can be facilitated if certain features are assessed (Table 45.3).

Distal myopathy with rimmed vacuoles (Nonaka myopathy; hereditary inclusion body myopathy,

Table 45.2. Distal myopathies with known gene defect

Name of myopathy	Gene/protein	Inheri-tance	Onset	First weakness
Tibial muscular dystrophy (Udd myopathy)	TTN/titin	AD	(Late) adulthood	Ankle dorsiflexors
Distal myotilinopathy	TTID/myotilin	AD	Late adulthood	Ankle plantar- and dorsiflexors
ZASPopathy (Markesbery–Griggs)	LDB3/ZASP	AD	Late adulthood	Ankle dorsiflexors
Matrin3 distal myopathy (VCPDM, MPD2)	MATR3/matrin3	AD	Late adulthood	Ankle dorsiflexors or finger extensors; also vocal cord and pharyngeal weakness
VCP-mutated distal myopathy	VCP/VCP	AD	Late adulthood	Variable
Alpha-B crystallin mutated distal myopathy	CRYAB/aB-crystallin	AD	(Late) adulthood	Variable
Distal caveolinopathy	CAV3/caveolin	AD	(Early) adulthood	Small hand muscles
Desminopathy	Des/desmin	AD	(Early) adulthood	Ankle dorsiflexion
Distal ABD-filaminopathy	FLNC/FLNC	AD	(Early) adulthood	Finger flexors
Laing distal myopathy (MPD1)	MYH7/Beta-MyHHC	AD	(Early) childhood	Finger and wrist extensors, ankle and hallux dorsiflexors, neck flexors
KLHL9 mutated distal myopathy	KLHL9/KLHL9	AD	(Early) childhood	Ankle dorsiflexors
Distal nebulin myopathy	NEB/nebulin	AR	Childhood	Finger and wrist extensors, ankle dorsiflexors
Miyoshi myopathy (MM1)	DYSF/dysferlin	AR	Early adulthood	Ankle plantar flexors
Distal anoctaminopathy (MMD3)	ANO5/anoctamin-5	AR	Adulthood	Ankle plantar flexors
Distal myopathy with rimmed vacuoles (Nonaka)	GNE/GNE	AR	Early adulthood	Ankle and toe dorsiflexors

As more patients with distal myopathies are being recognized, the variation of phenotypes will increase.

In this book we have focused upon patients who experienced first manifestations during late adolescence or in adulthood. Diseases that manifest in children have been included for completeness; www.musclegenetable.fr; www.neuromuscular.wustl.edu

Table 45.3. What to assess if a diagnosis of hereditary distal myopathy is suspected

- Mode of inheritance
- Age at onset
- Affected muscle groups (anterior versus posterior muscles of the leg, and upper versus lower limb muscles)
- Presence of cardiac involvement
- Activity of serum creatine kinase
- Histopathological abnormalities: dystrophic features, myofibrillar disorganization, and rimmed vacuoles (can be absent in myofibrillar myopathies)

GNE-pathy) usually presents in the late teens or early adulthood with progressive weakness of foot and toe dorsiflexors causing notable foot drop and steppage gait. Weakness shows distal to proximal progression with relative sparing of the quadriceps femoris muscles, often leading to loss of ambulation. Rehabilitation medicine plays an important role in the management of these patients. Serum CK activity is normal or moderately increased. Muscle biopsy specimens show rimmed vacuoles, and at later stages, dystrophic changes.

Suggested reading

Gidaro T, Morosetti R, Mirabella M. Hereditary inclusion-body myopathy: clues on pathogenesis and possible therapy. *Muscle Nerve* 2009; **40**: 340–349.

Malicdan MC, Nonaka I. Distal myopathies, a review: highlights on distal myopathies with rimmed vacuoles. *Neurol India* 2008; **56**: 314–324.

Mastaglia FL, Lamont PJ, Laing NG. Distal myopathies. *Curr Opin Neurol* 2005; **18**: 504–510.

Udd B. Distal myopathies–new genetic entities expand diagnostic challenge. *Neuromusc Disord* 2012; **22**: 5–12.

Oculopharyngeal muscular dystrophy: an elderly woman denying difficulties swallowing

Clinical history

A 68-year-old woman was referred because of slowly progressive difficulties climbing stairs. Four years earlier she had had ptosis surgery. Her mother had been diagnosed with progressive external ophthalmoplegia at the age of 69 years. She denied having swallowing difficulties, but her daughter stressed that eating biscuits took her mother much more time than others.

Examination

There was symmetric ptosis and a minor limitation of eye movements without diplopia. There was no dysarthria and no weakness of neck muscles. Finger extensors, hip abductors, and foot dorsal flexors were slightly weak. She had no problems getting up from a chair. Gait was slightly waddling.

Ancillary investigations

DNA analysis showed an expansion of the number of (GCG) trinucleotide repeats in the polyadenylate binding nuclear 1 (PABPN1) gene (n=16, normal n=10). This finding is diagnostic for OPMD.

Diagnostic considerations

The combination of ptosis, dysphagia, and familial occurrence makes OPMD a likely diagnosis. Limitation of eye movements is not an early sign in OPMD, but may occur in elderly patients. Diplopia is not a prominent complaint.

Mitochondrial disease is an alternative diagnosis in a patient with slowly progressive, symmetric external ophthalmoplegia without diplopia. Initially, difficulties with swallowing were denied by this patient, probably because she had unconsciously adapted by chewing her food thoroughly.

General remarks

OPMD is a rare, slowly progressive disease of skeletal muscles, notably the levator palpebrae and pharyngeal muscles. Onset is usually in the fifth decade with ptosis and dysphagia. In later stages limb muscles may also become weak (Figure 46.1). Males and females are equally affected. Life expectancy of OPMD is normal. In old age, ambulation may become impaired. There is no cardiac involvement. Inheritance is AD with complete penetrance in most families.

The cause is a GCG-triplet expansion in the first exon of the PABPN1 gene on chromosome 14.q11.1. The effects of the resulting lengthening of the PABPN1 polyalanine domain are as yet speculative, and may involve impaired function of mRNA and accumulation of undegradable material forming nuclear filamentous inclusions. The triplet repeat in PABPN1 is stable in contrast to other (polyglutamine) triplet disorders (Case 5). There is no known clinical anticipation in OPMD.

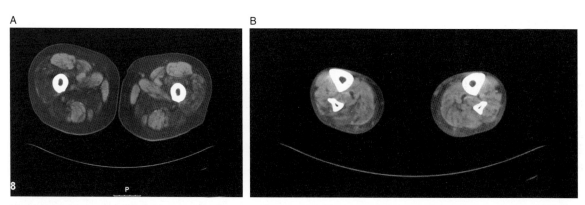

Figure 46.1. CT scan at the level of the upper leg shows severely abnormal lateral and medial vastus muscles with sparing of the rectus femoris muscles. The biceps femoris muscles are also severely affected. The gastrocnemius muscles have disappeared, whereas the soleus muscles have been relatively spared. (B).

Table 46.1. Dysphagia in adult patients with neuromuscular disease

- The most dangerous complications are choking and consequent respiratory tract infections, and weight loss (e.g., ALS)
- Dysphagia can be a prominent feature of many other neuromuscular diseases: GBS, myasthenia gravis, DM type 1, OPMD, IBM
- Many patients with chronic disease will adapt their eating style and diet (e.g., patients with ALS do not tend to empty their plate)
- >10% weight loss can be an indication for percutaneous endoscopic gastrostomy
- Consult ear–nose–throat specialist for diagnostic tests in patients with chronic muscle disease (videofluoroscopy with modified barium swallow)
- Interventions include dietary modifications, swallowing maneuvers and surgical interventions; e.g., cricopharyngeal myotomy
- There is no current evidence for choice of the most appropriate treatment for an individual

Management of a patient with OPMD may include ptosis surgery and advice on swallowing technique and diet. Cricopharyngeal myotomy and percutaneous gastrostomy may also be considered (Table 46.1).

Suggested reading

Abu-Baker A, Rouleau GA. Oculopharyngeal muscular dystrophy: recent advances in the understanding of the molecular pathogenic mechanisms and treatment strategies. *Biochim Biophys Acta* 2007; **1772**: 173–185.

Brais B. Oculopharyngeal muscular dystrophy: a late-onset polyalanine disease. *Cytogenet Genome Res* 2003; **100**: 252–260.

Hill M, Hughes T, Milford C. Treatment for swallowing difficulties (dysphagia) in chronic muscle disease. *Cochrane Database Syst Rev* 2004; **2**: CD004303.

Van der Sluijs BM, Hoefsloot LH, Padberg GW, van der Maarel SV, van Engelen BGM. Oculopharyngeal muscular dystrophy with limb girdle weakness as major complaint. *J Neurol* 2003; **250**: 1307–1312.

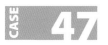

Myofibrillar myopathies: desminopathy: a woman with a family history of muscle weakness and severe cardiac complaints, desminopathy

Clinical history

A 36-year-old woman was concerned about being affected with an autosomal dominantly inherited disease that runs in the family. A few years before presentation, she had noticed difficulty when walking in the mountains and this had gradually progressed to difficult climbing stairs and an inability to run. She also noted that she could no longer lift her head when in the supine position. Her mother had died from this disease in her early forties. She knew that many affected family members had been diagnosed with cardiac arrhythmias and cardiac conduction abnormalities in addition to muscle weakness. Some were treated with an implantable cardioverter defibrillator. In elderly family members, cardiac enlargement was not uncommon.

Examination

On examination, VC was 81% of expected. There was a slight dysarthria, and a moderate weakness of neck flexors and hip and knee flexors. There were positive Gowers' and Trendelenburg signs and she could not walk on her heels.

Ancillary investigations

Serum CK was mildly increased. Light and electron microscopic examination of muscle biopsies in this family had shown disruption of the myofibrillar organization and accumulation of granulofilamentous material (Figure 47.1). DNA analysis of the desmin gene showed the p.Asn342Asp mutation.

Diagnostic considerations

In patients with AD inherited axial-proximal-distal distribution of weakness and cardiac involvement, it is justified to start the diagnostic work-up with analysis of the desmin gene. A diagnosis of desminopathy, one of the myofibrillar myopathies could be made.

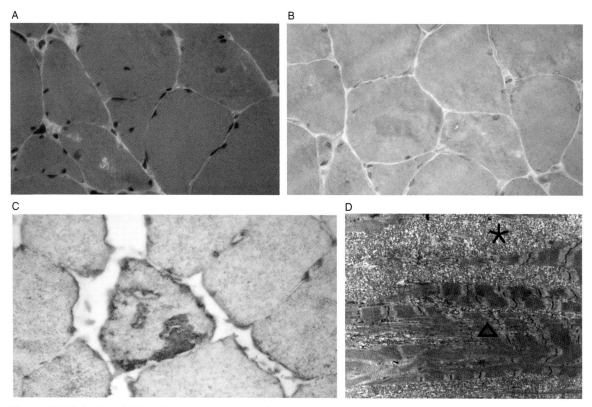

Figure 47.1. Skeletal muscle biopsy showing variation in muscle fiber size with small vacuoles and accumulation of eosinophilic material in the hematoxylin and eosin (HE) staining (A), that is more obvious in the modified Gomori trichrome staining (B). The diffuse and single inclusions contain desmin (C). (D) (electronmicrograph) shows granulofilamentous material (asterisk) that is interspersed among disorganized myofibrils (triangle).

Follow-up

Five years after presentation she could only just walk independently. VC had decreased to 70% in the sitting position and 52% when lying down; e.g., postural drop. A year later, she experienced frequent anxious night-time awakenings and headaches on waking in the morning. During the day she felt tired. Nocturnal measurements of pCO_2 showed an abnormal increase. Consequently, nocturnal noninvasive ventilatory support was initiated causing her to feel much better. Asymptomatic ventricular tachycardia and right bundle branch block were diagnosed. Four years later, she became wheelchair-dependent and lost ambulation completely.

General remarks

The myobrillar myopathies are defined on the basis of their histopathological abnormalities. The most characteristic feature is best identified on electron microscopy and consists of disorganization of the sarcomere, starting at the Z-disk. Degraded granulofilamentous material accumulates between myofibrils and membranous organelles, and glycogen aggregates in autophagic vacuoles. Accumulating proteins include desmin, dystrophin, and beta-amyloid precursor protein.

Despite these distinctive features, it can be difficult to make a diagnosis of myofibrillar myopathy, because at the light microscopic level, these abnormalities may be difficult to recognize or can be overlooked if not abundantly present. Routine examination of a muscle biopsy specimen can show many rather aspecific features, such as degeneration and regeneration, necrosis and increased fibrosis (suggesting muscular dystrophy), vacuoles and grouped atrophy, and abnormal protein aggregates appearing as amorphous, granular, or hyaline deposits in various shapes, colors, and localizations (in frozen sections).

In addition, the clinical presentation is variable. Progressive distal muscle weakness of the legs is often the first symptom, but patients can also show a limb girdle or scapuloperoneal distribution of weakness. Respiratory insufficiency, axial weakness, facial weakness, dysphagia, and dysarthria also occur. Cardiac involvement is frequent and cardiac evaluation should thus be part of the diagnostic work-up of any myopathy with dystrophic features or intrafiber structural abnormalities (see Table 38.1). Myofibrillar myopathies are AD inherited in most families.

At the molecular genetic level, all mutations found to cause myofibrillar myopathy to date involve Z-disk-associated proteins, in particular desmin, and also alphaB-crystallin, myotilin, ZASP, filamin C, and Bag3. Mutation analysis is becoming more and more available as part of the routine diagnostic work-up in myofibrillar myopathies.

Desmin is an intermediate filament necessary for the structural integrity of all types of muscle cells. Most patients with a desminopathy present in their teens or adulthood with progressive weakness in a distal, limb girdle or scapuloperoneal pattern. These different phenotypes can coexist within one family. Skeletal weakness in desminopathy is often accompanied by cardiomyopathy resulting in chronic heart failure and cardiac conduction failure, leading to conduction blocks, arrhythmias, and sudden death. Cardiac involvement may be the only sign of desminopathy. Management of a patient with a desminopathy includes genetic counseling, rehabilitation medicine, regular cardiac examinations, and symptomatic treatment. Cardiac examination should also be offered to asymptomatic, at-risk relatives of a patient with a desminopathy. The inheritance pattern of desminopathy is usually AD but can be AR. Many sporadic cases are caused by de novo mutations.

Suggested reading

Goldfarb LG, Dalakas MC. Tragedy in a heartbeat: malfunctioning desmin causes skeletal and cardiac muscle disease. *J Clin Invest* 2009; **119**: 1806–1813.

Olivé M, Odgerel Z, Martínez A, et al. Clinical and myopathological evaluation of early- and late-onset subtypes of myofibrillar myopathy. *Neuromuscul Disord* 2011; **21**: 533–542.

Selcen D. Myofibrillar myopathies. *Neuromuscul Disord* 2011; **21**: 161–171.

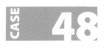

Late-onset congenital myopathy caused by a mutation in the RYR1 gene, central core disease: a nurse with tired legs

Clinical history

For the past 15 years, a 36-year-old nurse had increasingly felt tired legs. Although she could walk normally on flat surfaces, she could run only a few steps. Walking uphill was also tiring. When climbing stairs she needed the banister to remain stable. Because of the tiredness she changed jobs and became a pharmacist's assistant.

At the age of 7 years, she had had surgery for habitual patellar luxation, and when she was 17 years old, for short Achilles tendons. At school she was a member of a gymnastics club and had no problems in keeping up with her peers at sport. The family history was negative. The parents were unrelated.

Examination

She had atrophic calves, "hollow" feet, and hammer toes. Manual muscle testing showed no weakness, but she needed her arms when rising from the squatting position. The knee reflexes were hypoactive and the Achilles tendon reflexes were absent. She could not walk on her heels. Trendelenburg sign was absent. She had no scoliosis.

Ancillary investigations

CK activity ranged between 277 and 632 U/L (1.6–3.7 ULN). EMG of the anterior tibial and rectus femoris muscles showed polyphasic amplitudes. The muscle CT scan was severely abnormal (Figure 48.1). A biopsy of the deltoid muscle showed multiple cores (Figure 48.2). Exon 40 of one and exon 93 of the other ryanodine receptor 1 (RYR1) genes had pathogenic mutations. The missense c.6617C>T (pThr2206Met) mutation in exon 40 has previously been associated with malignant hyperthermia.

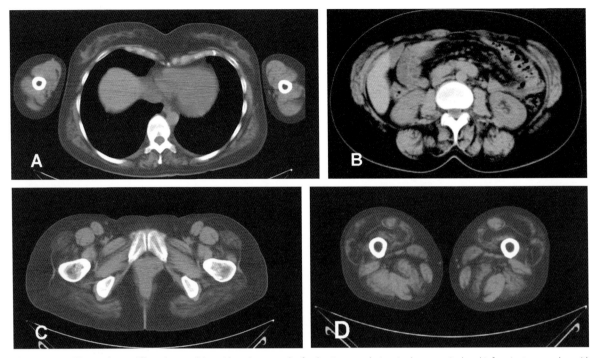

Figure 48.1. CT scan shows diffuse abnormalities with replacement by fat that is most obvious in the paraspinal and infraspinatus muscles, with relative sparing of the biceps and triceps brachii muscles (A), abdominal wall and paraspinal muscles (B), gluteus and quadriceps femoris muscles (C), and in almost all muscles at the level of the middle of the thigh, with relative sparing of the biceps femoris, gracilis, and sartorius muscles (D).

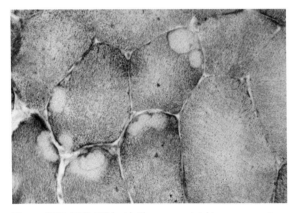

Figure 48.2. NADH-TR (oxidative enzyme stain) transverse section from the deltoid muscle biopsy shows numerous cores of varying size at the periphery of the muscle fibers. Cores occur more frequently in oxidative type 1 muscle fibers. In most cases, the cores are of the structured type, that is, they retain a degree of striated myofibrillar pattern and myofibrillar ATPase activity.

Diagnostic considerations and follow-up

A diagnosis of central core disease was made. As the patient was a compound heterozygote, she could be informed that her children were carriers of one mutated RYR1 gene, but unlikely to develop similar complaints. However, she and her offspring with a mutation in exon 40 were at risk of developing malignant hyperthermia when receiving general anesthetics and muscle relaxants. She was referred to the rehabilitation physician for advice on work and physical activity.

General remarks

This patient had the following features: onset in the second decade of life, patellar luxation and foot deformities, mild proximal muscle weakness of the lower limbs, and exercise intolerance. CK elevation was mild. Muscle imaging showed prominent abnormalities. The referring neurologist excluded SMA type 3, Kugelberg–Welander disease, by DNA analysis of the SMN gene (Case 6). We excluded Pompe disease. Congenital myasthenia gravis was unlikely because of the CK elevation. Other differential diagnostic possibilities included carriership of DMD muscular dystrophy, one of the LGMDs, mitochondrial myopathy, and late-onset congenital myopathy. Most of these diseases can be further diagnosed through a skeletal muscle biopsy.

Congenital myopathies usually have their onset in infancy, or antenatally with a decrease in fetal movement. In some patients, onset is in the second decade or even in adulthood. Skeletal muscle biopsies show characteristic abnormalities that can lead to a diagnosis of congenital fiber disproportion, central core disease, multiminicore disease, centronuclear myopathy, myofibrillar myopathy, or nemalin myopathy. Causative genes are becoming identified increasingly, as is greater variation in phenotype.

Central core disease is a relatively mild congenital myopathy, usually characterized by delayed motor milestones and mild proximal weakness of the legs. Rarely, there is predominant weakness of paraspinal muscles, especially in late-onset cases. Orthopedic complications include congenital dislocation of the hips, scoliosis, and foot deformities. Patients with central core disease are at risk of malignant hyperthermia. The skeletal muscle biopsy is characterised by multiple cores or areas of absent oxidative enzyme activity due to mitochondrial depletion. Typically, cores run along a longitudinal stretch of the muscle fiber.

Most cases of central core disease are due to mutations in the RYR1 gene. Most patients have autosomal dominant inheritance with autosomal recessive inheritance, usually heterozygous, occurring in a minority. The large RYR1 gene encodes for a protein that functions as the principal sarcoplasmic reticulum calcium release channel regulating Ca^{2+} content in skeletal muscle during excitation–contraction coupling. RYR-1 mutations cause a lower activation threshold.

Dominant RYR1 mutations, associated with typical central core disease, cluster in a mutational hotspot affecting the C-terminus. In addition, RYR1 gene mutations are associated with late-onset axial myopathy, multiminicore disease, and centronuclear myopathy.

Malignant hyperthermia is a pharmacogenetic disorder in which susceptible patients develop generalized muscle contracture followed by a hypermetabolic state with high fever. Rhabdomyolysis may follow. The drugs involved, inhaled general anesthetics or the depolarizing muscle relaxant, succinylcholine, lead to massive calcium release from the sarcoplasmic reticulum. Malignant hyperthermia susceptibility is analyzed using in vitro contracture tests (www.emhg.org). Mutations associated with malignant hyperthermia are distributed throughout the RYR1 coding sequence.

Suggested reading

Jungbluth H, Lillis S, Zhou H, et al. Late-onset axial myopathy with cores due to a novel heterozygous dominant mutation in the skeletal muscle ryanodine receptor 1 (RYR1) gene. *Neuromusc Disord* 2009; **19**: 344–347.

Klingler W, Rueffert H, Lehmann-Horn F, Girard T, Hopkins PM. Core myopathies and risk of malignant hyperthermia. *Anaesth Analg* 2009; **109**; 1167–1173.

Wu S, Ibarra CA, Christine M, et al. Central core disease is due to RYR1 mutations in more than 90% of patients. *Brain* 2006; **129**: 1470–1480.

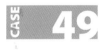

CASE 49 — Bethlem myopathy: a laborer manifesting with muscle contractures

Clinical history

A 55-year-old patient had had muscle complaints for as long as he could remember. He could not stretch his arms, or walk without shoes due to deformities of the feet. His power endurance was low, but he still worked full-time as a manual worker. He was otherwise healthy.

Family history revealed that his father was similarly affected. In addition, a half-brother and half-sister not only had contractures but also muscle weakness. The latter underwent surgery for torticollis in the neonatal period.

Examination

There were flexion contractures of the elbows, contractures of the wrists and knees, and shortening of the Achilles tendons (Figure 49.1). He had pes cavus and claw toes.

Atrophy of the sternocleidomastoid muscle was observed, and there was slight weakness of the neck

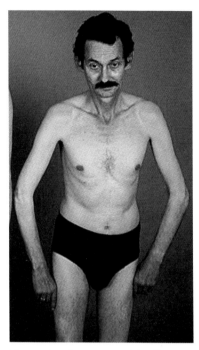

Figure 49.1. Contractures of the elbows in a patient with Bethlem myopathy.

flexors, infraspinatus, triceps brachii, and iliopsoas muscles.

Ancillary investigations

Serum CK activity was normal. A heterozygous missense mutation (c.739-1G>A) was found in the collagen VI, COL6A1 gene.

Diagnostic considerations

Proximal muscle weakness was mild and slowly progressive over years, and contractures had always been prominent. Combined with the probable AD inheritance, these features suggested Bethlem myopathy, or Emery–Dreifuss muscular dystrophy due to mutations in the emerin gene, or in the lamin A/C gene (Case 42).

The only distinctive features are torticollis in Bethlem myopathy, and heart involvement in the Emery–Dreifuss muscular dystrophies caused by emerin or lamin A/C mutations. No heart involvement was found in our patient. DNA analysis on Bethlem myopathy was carried out based on the presence of torticollis in his sibling.

General remarks

In 1976, the neurologists Jaap Bethlem and George van Wijngaarden, who worked in the University Hospital in Amsterdam, reported Bethlem myopathy as a "Benign myopathy, with autosomal dominant inheritance" in three Dutch pedigrees. Subsequently, a linkage was found between Bethlem myopathy and the COL6A1-COL62 gene complex localized on chromosome 21. Shortly thereafter, linkage was detected with the COL6A3 gene on chromosome 2. This paved the way for the identification of mutations in these three genes encoding three subunits, peptide chains that form type VI collagen, and a ubiquitous extracellular matrix protein capable of forming an interstitial and pericellular microfibrillar network. As this network is closely associated with the basement membrane around skeletal muscle fibers, collagen VI plays a role in the integrity and function of the skeletal muscle. This notion of extracellular dysfunction explains why contractures form an early and predominant part of the spectrum of Bethlem myopathy.

There is great variation in the manifestation of Bethlem myopathy, even within families. In our patient, muscle contractures were the predominant feature and his half-sister also exhibited muscle weakness and torticollis. Other patients may have had diminished fetal movements, or have been born as floppy babies with extension contractures of the feet that resolved spontaneously. Children with limb girdle distribution of muscle weakness with hyperlaxity of the knee joints have also been reported. In the classic type of patient, life expectancy is usually normal. After the age of 60 years, a fair proportion of patients has to use walking aids or a wheelchair for outdoor transportation. In about 10% of the cases, respiratory insufficiency occurs due to involvement of the diaphragm. The heart is not affected.

The combination of muscle weakness, hyperlaxity, and contractures is also present in Ullrich congenital muscular dystrophy, which runs a more progressive course with early scoliosis and respiratory insufficiency. This resemblance to Bethlem myopathy led to the discovery that collagen VI mutations were also the culprit in this condition, whose inheritance was long considered to be AR. Genetic counseling is not, however, straightforward, as over the past decade, severe cases with AD inheritance and relatively mild cases of AR inheritance have been described. Thus, classic Bethlem myopathy and Ullrich congenital muscular dystrophy are now considered to be at opposite ends of a phenotypic spectrum. Phenotypic variability can in part be explained by the extent to which the mutant collagen protein can participate in the collagen VI assembly.

Suggested reading

Bethlem J, Wijngaarden GK. Benign myopathy with autosomal dominant inheritance. A report on three pedigrees. *Brain* 1976; **99**: 91–100.

Jöbsis GJ, Boers JM, Barth PG, de Visser M. Bethlem myopathy: a slowly progressive congenital muscular dystrophy with contractures. *Brain* 1999; **122**: 649–655.

Lampe AK, Bushby KM. Collagen VI related muscle disorders. *J Med Genet* 2005; **42**: 673–685.

Lampe AK, Zou Y, Sudano D, et al. Exon skipping mutations in collagen VI are common and are predictive for severity and inheritance. *Hum Mutat* 2008; **29**: 809–822.

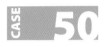

CASE 50

Myotonic dystrophy type 1, Curschmann–Steinert disease: a man with no complaints

Clinical history

A 29-year-old electrotechnician was referred by a dental surgeon who treated him for dysgnathia. He suspected DM because of impaired speech and painless, short-lasting stiffness in the hands after using them with force. Speech had gradually become less clear during the previous years. Otherwise, he hardly mentioned symptoms apart from the loss of hair. His father had developed frontal balding from the age of 30.

Examination

On examination, there was frontotemporal baldness and atrophy of temporal muscles (See Introduction, Figure 13). Myotonia could be easily elicited in the hands and tongue. There was bulbar dysarthria and slight weakness of foot dorsal flexor muscles.

Ancillary investigations

On DNA analysis of the dystrophia myotonica protein kinase (DMPK) gene, there was one normal allele (CTG repeats <50) and one allele with an expanded number (399) of CTG repeats.

ECG was normal; 24-hour registration of the cardiac rhythm revealed no disturbances. A typical cataract was found on split-lamp examination.

Diagnostic considerations

The combination of bulbar dysarthria, premature balding, and myotonia are diagnostic for DM. DNA analysis to confirm the diagnosis is relatively easy.

Follow-up

During the subsequent years, he received standardized check-ups by a trained nurse who coordinated multidisciplinary care by the family doctor, neurologist, cardiologist, pulmonologist, ophthalmologist, gastroenterologist, geneticist, and rehabilitation services. Atrium flutter was treated by medication and later, atrium fibrillation was treated by electrocardioversion. Belches and diarrhea improved using movicolon. He was treated for pneumonia, probably following choking. VC decreased to 64% of the value predicted on the basis of height and age, but there were no signs of nocturnal hypercapnia or hypnea. He was instructed to use airstacking because of decreased coughing force in order to prevent further infections. Weakness increased fairly quickly, especially of distal muscles. Walking devices secured ambulation. Soon after the diagnosis had been made, he lost his job and became increasingly passive. His wife could not cope and the couple accepted psychological assistance. After preimplantation diagnostic procedures, a healthy son was born.

General remarks

DM type 1 is the most common type of muscular dystrophy and the most common myotonic disorder in adults, with an estimated prevalence worldwide of 5–20 per 100 000. The disease is AD inherited. DM1 results from the unstable expansion of cytosine–thymine–guanine (CTG) trinucleotide repeats in the 3′ untranslated region of the DMPK gene on chromosome 19. Genetic anticipation refers to a more severe and earlier onset phenotype in the subsequent generation, secondary to an increase in the repeat size. The congenital form of DM1 results from a CTG repeat

143

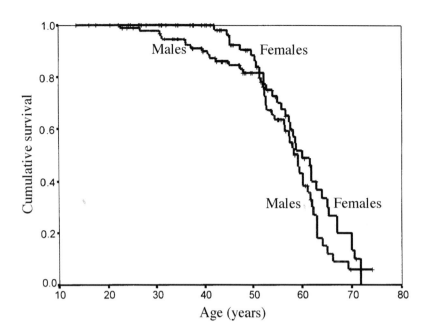

Figure 50.1. Kaplan–Meier survival curves of adult-onset DM patients (n=180) showing that half of the patients had died by the age of 60 years; 60% of the deceased patients had died of pneumonia or cardiac arrhythmia. (From De Die-Smulders CEM, Höweler CJ, Thijs C, et al. Age and causes of death in adult-onsetmyotonic dystrophy. *Brain* 1998; **121**: 1557–1563, with permission.)

increase from a few hundred base pairs in an affected mother to several thousand base pairs in the ovum.

The clinical diagnosis of DM can easily be made from the characteristic combination of symptoms and signs. Myotonia can usually be demonstrated clinically or electrophysiologically, but generally does not result in disability (Video 1). Patients have prominent wasting and weakness of superficial facial muscles, levator palpebrae superioris, temporalis, masseter, and palate muscles with resultant ptosis, dysarthria, and loss of facial expression (see Figure 13). Swallowing may be impaired early in the disease. Sternocleidomastoid and distal muscles in the extremities are preferentially involved. Owing to distal weakness of the legs, patients may walk with bilateral foot drop or mild steppage gait (Video 1).

Diaphragm weakness may result in life-threatening hypoventilation. Cardiac involvement, in the form of conduction delay, atrial flutter and fibrillation, and subsequent cardiomyopathy is common (see Table 38.1). Sudden cardiac death, presumably related to arrhythmia, is a major and preventable cause of mortality. Pneumonia is another major cause of premature death (Figure 50.1).

A characteristic cataract before the age of 40 years is another common feature. Cataract can be present without skeletal muscle or cardiac disease and may lead to a new diagnosis of DM in a pedigree. CNS disease characterized by apathy, somnolence, and inertia leads to psychological and social impairments. Other systemic manifestations include gastrointestinal problems, frontal balding (see Introduction, Figure 13), testicular atrophy, hypogammaglobulinemia, and insulin resistance.

DM patients frequently do not report symptoms. Many neuromuscular centers, therefore, support their patients by regular multidisciplinary screening enabling timely symptomatic treatment and counseling. This should include recognition of the burden experienced by the partner and family.

Without supportive treatment, patients with DM1 die at a younger age than expected. Arrhythmia may require pacemaker or cardioverter-defibrillator implantation. Nocturnal hypoventilation and obstructive and central apneas are causes of excessive day-time sleepiness (EDS). Noninvasive assisted ventilation during the night may substantially improve the quality of life. Modafinil may be tried to treat EDS if there is no evidence of sleep-disordered breathing. Gastrointestinal problems, especially diarrhea, can be disabling, and should be treated accordingly. Special attention should be given to cognitive, emotional, and behavioral problems in children. Genetic counseling should be offered. Prenatal diagnostic testing is available.

Suggested reading

Cup EH, Kinebanian A, Satink T, et al. Living with myotonic dystrophy; what can be learned from couples? A qualitative study. *BMC Neurol* 2011; **11**: 86–98.

Turner C, Hilton-Jones D. The myotonic dystrophies: diagnosis and management. *J Neurol Neurosurg Psychiatry* 2010; **81**: 358–367.

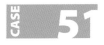

Myotonic dystrophy type 2, proximal myotonic myopathy: a woman with late-onset muscle weakness and syncope

Clinical history

A 60-year-old woman was referred because she had muscle weakness that led to increasing difficulty climbing stairs from the age of 50 years. In addition, she complained about exercise-induced myalgia.

Her previous history included cataract surgery at the age of 58 years, and lately, unexpected and unexplained falls. Family history revealed that several paternal family members were known to have early onset cataract. Her father had died suddenly and unexpectedly as did her brother, despite a pacemaker.

Examination

There was mild muscle weakness with a limb girdle distribution, the thighs were slightly atrophic, and the calf muscles firm. Gowers' phenomenon was positive. She had no facial weakness or diplegia. Myotonia could not be elicited. Reflexes were normal and there were no contractures.

Additional investigations

Serum CK activity was slightly elevated. EMG showed signs of myopathy, but no myotonia.

DNA analysis showed a CCTG repeat expansion of the one allele of the ZNF9 gene. Cardiac evaluation was abnormal.

Table 51.1. Features that discriminate myotonic dystrophy type 2 from type 1

- Milder disease course
- More prominent myalgia, stiffness, and fatigue
- Proximal muscle weakness
- Less weakness of the face and less bulbar weakness
- Frequent calf hypertrophy
- Apparent lack of mental retardation in juvenile cases
- Rarely congenital DM2
- Anticipation less pronounced

Diagnostic considerations

The combination of late-onset muscle weakness, cataract, and familial death due to a cardiac cause/involvement is consistent with a diagnosis of DM type 2 (previously called proximal myotonic myopathy, PROMM).

Once the diagnosis had been established, the cardiologist implanted a reveal cardiac monitor because of previous syncopes and her family history.

General remarks

The phenotype of DM2 resembles adult-onset DM1 as muscle weakness, myotonia, cataracts, and cardiac involvement occur in both, but differences exist (Table 51.1). Both are progressive multisystem disorders. In comparison to DM1, the degree of muscle weakness and atrophy is typically mild until late in the course of the disease.

The onset of DM2 is usually in the third decade of life, with muscle weakness being the most common presenting symptom. Most DM2 patients complain of more prominent muscle pain, stiffness, and fatigue compared to DM1 patients. The weakness in DM2 typically affects proximal muscles, including the neck, and elbow extensor and hip flexor muscles. In contrast, initial muscle involvement of DM1 tends to affect distal upper limb muscles. Patients with DM2 have less symptomatic distal, facial, and bulbar weakness, and less pronounced clinical myotonia.

Other clinical features include cardiac conduction defects, dilated cardiomyopathy (see Table 38.1), and posterior subcapsular cataracts that increase with age. Endocrine features are insulin insensitivity that increases with age and testicular failure. Cognitive manifestations in DM2 may include problems with organization, concentration, and word-finding. Excessive daytime sleepiness is less common.

Heredity is AD. The mutation that underlies DM2 is a CCTG repeat expansion in intron 1 of zinc finger protein 9 on chromosome 3q.

Suggested reading

Day JW, Jacobsen F, Rasmussen LJ, et al. Myotonic dystrophy type 2: molecular, diagnostic and clinical spectrum. *Neurology* 2003; **60**: 657–664.

Schoser BG, Ricker K, Schneider-Gold C, et al. Sudden cardiac death in myotonic dystrophy type 2. *Neurology* 2004; **63**: 2402–2404.

Turner C, Hilton-Jones D. The myotonic dystrophies: diagnosis and management. *J Neurol Neurosurg Psychiatry* 2010; **81**: 358–367.

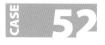

CASE 52 — Becker myotonia, chloride channelopathy: a buyer in search of medication for his muscle stiffness

Clinical history

A 35-year-old male complained about muscle stiffness and weakness, especially at the start of a movement. He had experienced these symptoms for as long as he could remember. They were present in his eyes, jaws, tongue, and limb muscles. He had noticed that cold weather had a negative influence. In spite of these symptoms, he experienced no limitations in activities of daily living. He was referred because he had been informed elsewhere about possible treatment. The family history revealed similar symptoms in his two siblings. His parents were consanguineous. His father's grandparents were cousins.

Examination

He had hypertrophy of the calf muscles and of the quadriceps femoris muscle. When asked to open his eyes after first firmly closing them, we observed action myotonia of the orbicularis oculi muscle that consisted of not being able to open the eyes (Figure 52.1). When he made a fist he had action myotonia of the hand muscles. There was percussion myotonia of various limb muscles.

When setting off, his gait was stiff; this gradually improved as the muscles "warmed up." Similarly, he noticed weakness of the neck flexors and of various arm and leg muscles, which also improved after sustained contraction of the muscles. He was found to have a lumbar hyperlordosis and slight contractures at the elbows and wrists. Arm reflexes were normal whereas the knee jerks were decreased and Achilles tendon reflexes absent.

Ancillary investigations

DNA analysis revealed that he was a compound heterozygote with a missense mutation in exon 8 and an unclassified variant in exon 17 of the chloride channel (CLCN1) gene located on chromosome 7q35.

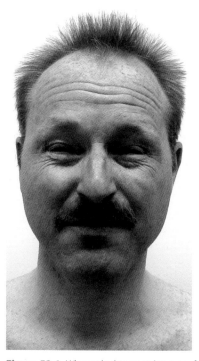

Figure 52.1. When asked to open his eyes after first firmly closing them, action myotonia of the orbicularis oculi muscle was observed, which resulted in not being able to open the eyes properly.

Diagnostic considerations and follow-up

The patient had two key features that led to the diagnosis of nondystrophic myotonia: episodic muscle weakness and a "warm up" phenomenon; e.g., decrease of myotomia with continuing exercise. The diagnosis was refined by DNA analysis, which showed that the patient was suffering from an autosomal recessive form of myotonia, also called Becker myotonia.

General remarks

Nondystrophic myotonic syndromes comprise a heterogeneous group of skeletal muscle disorders caused by

Table 52.1. Clinical features of the nondystrophic myotonias

	AR myotonia congenita (Becker)	AD myotonia congenita (Thomsen)	Paramyotonia congenita (Eulenburg)	Other sodium-channel myotonias
Causative gene	CLCN1	CLCN1	SCN4A	SCN4A
Onset	First decade	Infancy–adulthood	Infancy	First decade
Episodic muscle weakness	On initiation of movements. Rapid improvement on sustained muscle contraction	Mild, exercise- and pregnancy-related	After exercise, on exposure to cold, spontaneous	Absent
Warm-up phenomenon	Present	Present	Present	Present
Paradoxal and painful myotonia	Absent	Absent	Present	Can be present
Worsening of myotonia upon exposure to cold/cold-induced myotonia	Infrequent	Infrequent	Profound	Can be present
Most frequent distribution of myotonia	Muscles of hands and legs	Muscles of hands and legs	Muscles of the face, neck, and arms	Generalized
Muscle hypertrophy	Present	Present	Can be present	Can be present

Adapted from Matthews E, Fialho D, Tan SV, et al. The nondystrophic myotonias: molecular pathogenesis, diagnosis and treatment. *Brain* 2010; **133**; 9–22.
Paradoxal myotonia: myotonia that appears during exercise.
Myopathy may develop in some patients with nondystrophic myotonia. Permanent severe myopathy seems to be more common in patients with periodic paralysis.

mutations in genes encoding the skeletal muscle chloride (CLCN1) or sodium channels (SCN4A) (Table 52.1).

For those patients with mild symptoms, no specific drug treatment may be needed, although it is important to provide advice regarding the avoidance of precipitating factors such as exposure to cold or strenuous exercise. Various drugs have been tried and the class Ib anti-arrhythmic mexiletine a sodium channel blocker, which generally is considered to be the first-line treatment of choice by neuromuscular experts, is usually well tolerated with only minor side effects reported in dosages of 150–200 mg TID. Recently a randomized placebo-controlled, crossover trial showed that a four-week course of mexiletine caused improvement of stiffness compared to the placebo. The drug was safe and well tolerated.

Periodic paralysis

In addition to myotonia, sodium channel disorders may manifest with episodic proximal muscle weakness with onset in the first decade or later provoked by exercise, cold, pregnancy, fasting, steroids, and potassium loading. The attacks usually occur before breakfast, last 15 to 60 minutes, and are associated with high serum potassium levels, hyperkalemic periodic paralysis. Many attacks are brief and do not need treatment. Carbohydrate intake and mild exercise may offer relief.

Hypokalemic periodic paralysis, most frequently caused by mutations in the calcium channel gene, is characterized by attacks of proximal muscles weakness at night or early in the morning. Rhabdomyolysis occurs with specific mutations. Onset of the attacks is usually in the first or second decade and females are less affected. Provocative factors include carbohydrate-rich meals, rest after exercise, heat or cold, stress, and some drugs (steroids, insulin). Serum potassium is low during attacks. A muscle biopsy may show tubular aggregates and vacuoles.

Suggested reading

Matthews E, Fialho D, Tan SV, et al. The non-dystrophic myotonias: molecular pathogenesis, diagnosis and treatment. *Brain* 2010: **133**; 9–22.

Miller T, Dias da Silva MR, Miller HA. Correlating phenotype and genotype in the periodic paralyses. *Neurology* 2004; **63**: 1647–1655.

Stratland JM, Bundy BN, Wang Y, et al. Mexiletine for symptoms and signs of myotonia in nondystrophic myotonia: a randomised controlled trial. *JAMA* 2012; **308**: 1357–1365.

Trip J, Drost G, Ginjaar HB, **et al**. Redefining the clinical phenotypes of non-dystrophic myotonic syndromes. *J Neurol Neurosurg Psychiatry* 2009; **80**: 647–652.

Glycogen storage disease type 2, Pompe disease: a construction worker who could no longer carry a load while climbing a ladder

Clinical history

For the past two years, a 43-year-old construction worker has experienced progressive instability during work. When climbing a ladder with a load of tiles on his shoulder, he tended to fall backward. He had mild low back pain. A physical therapist noted hyperlordosis of the lumbar spine. Previously, his 45-year-old sister had been diagnosed with late-onset Pompe disease. She was wheelchair-dependent and received nocturnal noninvasive ventilation (NIV).

Examination

In a standing position, he had hyperlordosis. There was no skeletal muscle atrophy. He had mild scapular winging and mild weakness, MRC grade 4–5, of the hip flexor muscles. Otherwise, on testing, muscle strength was mostly normal, including strength of the paraspinal muscles when straightening up from a bent position. Gowers' sign was negative as he could rise from a squatting position without the help of his arms. He did, however, have to use his arms when sitting up from a supine position. He walked with his shoulders and arms held backwards (Video 21). When climbing stairs, he sometimes had to grasp the handrail. Knee tendon reflexes were absent.

Ancillary investigations

Serum CK activity was 11 × ULN (1700 U/L). VC was 105% of the expected value in the upright position. At the time, VC was not measured in the supine position. The CT scan of his muscular system was compatible with fatty degeneration of the abdominal wall and lumbar paraspinal muscles (Figure 53.1), and of the psoas and gluteus muscles with some abnormalities in the knee flexor muscles. Acid alpha-glucosidase (GAA), acid maltase, activity in leukocytes was decreased. He was found to be a compound heterozygote for Pompe disease with two mutations in the GAA gene: one 525delT severe, the other IVS 1–13 t>g with a mild effect.

Diagnostic considerations

The family history was positive for Pompe disease. The neurological examination showed postural abnormalities and weakness of the iliopsoas muscles. The ancillary tests confirmed the presence of a myopathy. Strictly speaking, measurement of GAA activity in leukocytes was not needed for a diagnosis as DNA analysis would have sufficed to confirm the diagnosis of Pompe disease. DNA analysis is indicated as other diseases may mimic Pompe disease.

Follow-up

Limb girdle type weakness gradually increased over the years. Although his condition stabilized with enzyme replacement therapy, he could not return to work. His VC remained stable.

General remarks

The patient was diagnosed with a mild form of late-onset Pompe disease. His symptoms were caused by weakness of the lower paraspinal muscles, which act to strengthen the spine, and by weakness of the hip flexors. These muscle groups need to reduce the angle of the hip joints when the center of gravity of the body is placed backward, as happens when climbing a ladder with a heavy weight on the shoulders.

Pompe disease, glycogen storage disease type 2 (GSD2), is a rare AR neuromuscular disease caused by deficiency of GAA, which degrades lysosomal glycogen. Patients are compound heterozygotes. Different mutations in the GAA gene lead to different residual degrees of GAA, and different rates of glycogen accumulation. A role for a disease modifying gene is hypothesized. The frequency of Pompe disease varies between one in 40 000 to one in 146 000 in different populations.

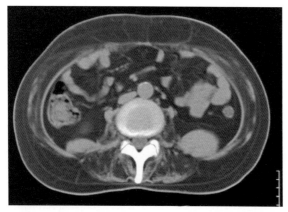

Figure 53.1. CT scan showing complete replacement by fat of the abdominal wall, erector trunci, and psoas major muscles (adjacent to the body of the vertebra).

Early onset, infantile Pompe disease manifests before birth with diminished movements of the child, or before the age of six months. Patients have two mutations with a severe pathogenic effect and GAA activity is virtually absent. Infants never sit or walk and have feeding difficulties. Ubiquitous glycogen storage leads to hepatomegaly, cardiomegaly, and macroglossia. Most infants die from cardiorespiratory failure before their first birthday.

Late-onset Pompe disease is caused by two mutations, one with a severe pathogenic effect, the other mild. A similar genotype may lead to variation of genotype between patients and in families. In the late-onset variant of Pompe disease, glycogen accumulation occurs only in skeletal muscle. The heart is not involved. Serum CK activity is elevated in almost all patients and may be as high as $10 \times$ ULN. Progression of weakness is slow over a period of years. Fatigue and muscle soreness are common initial complaints.

Most patients have symmetric limb girdle type of weakness and a varying degree of respiratory insufficiency. Lumbar lordosis occurs in 2/3 of patients, asymmetric scapular winging in 1/3, asymmetric ptosis and bulbar weakness in 1/4. Respiratory insufficiency from weakness of the diaphragm can be disproportional compared with limb muscle weakness. A postural drop is common (e.g., >10% decrease of VC in supine compared to the sitting position). Complaints of respiratory insufficiency are morning headaches and daytime fatigue.

For diagnostic purposes, a skeletal muscle biopsy is not always indicated. Adult patients with hyper-CK-emia with or without a chronic progressive limb girdle syndrome can be tested for GAA activity in leukocytes. If decreased, DNA testing may lead to a diagnosis of Pompe disease. Pompe disease can be strongly suspected if there are symptoms of respiratory insufficiency, or if postural drop exists. Usually, but deceivingly not always, a biopsy will reveal characteristic features (Figure 53.2).

The natural history of late-onset Pompe disease is characterized by slow, but unrelenting progression with a mean annual decline of VC in the upright seated position of 1%, and in the supine position of 1.3%. Declines in skeletal muscle strength and in respiratory function do not always occur at a similar pace. Respiratory function should be monitored at regular intervals. Pompe disease is the first treatable hereditary

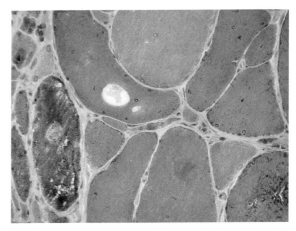

Figure 53.2. Modified Gomori trichrome stained transverse section of a vastus lateralis muscle biopsy of a patient with late-onset Pompe disease, showing increased variation of fiber size and increased number of internal nuclei. Most prominent are vacuoles that may contain eosinophilic material, which is also dispersed in the muscle fibers. With periodic acid Schiff staining, accumulation of glycogen in the muscle fibers was demonstrated (not shown).

myopathy. A recent trial with enzyme-replacement therapy (ERT) with biweekly intravenous GAA over an 18-month period showed improved walking distance and stabilization of pulmonary function. Without ERT, most adult patients finally require NIV and become wheelchair-dependent.

Suggested reading

Kroos M, Pomponio RJ, Van Vliet L, et al. Update of the Pompe disease mutation database with 107 sequence variants and a format for severity rating. *Hum Mutat* 2008; **29**: 13–26.

Van den Beek NAME, De Vries JM, Hagemans MLC, et al. The spectrum of Pompe disease: clinical features and prognostic factors for disease progression. *Orphanet J Rare Dis* [In Press].

Van der Ploeg A, Reuser A. Lysosomal storage disease 2. Pompe's disease. *Lancet* 2008; **372**: 1342–1353.

Van der Ploeg AT, Clemens PR, Corzo D, et al. A randomized study of alfaglucosidase alfa in late-onset Pompe's disease. *N Engl J Med* 2010; **363**: 1396–1406.

Wokke JHJ, Ausems MGEM, Van den Boogaard M-JH, et al. Genotype–phenotype correlation in adult-onset acid maltase deficiency. *Ann Neurol* 1995; **38**: 450–454.

Wokke JHJ, Escolar DM, Pestronk A, et al. Clinical features of late-onset Pompe's disease: a prospective cohort study. *Muscle Nerve* 2008; **38**: 1236–1245. www.pompecenter.nl.

Glycogen storage disease type 5, McArdle disease: a secretary with cramps in her hands who was found to have rhabdomyolysis

Clinical history

A 40-year-old female was referred because she had been complaining about cramping and swelling of the hands for more than four years. These symptoms bothered her when using her PC. She had never produced dark urine and she had never noticed muscle weakness. The previous disease history was inconspicuous except for goiter. The family history was negative for neuromuscular disorders.

Neurological examination

The neurological examination was normal.

Ancillary investigations

She was found to have a markedly elevated serum CK activity of >13 000 IU/L (>800 × ULN). Repeat measurement showed activities of 3389 and 1550 IU/L, respectively. The ischemic forearm test showed only a minimal increase in serum lactate (from a resting value of 0.4 to 0.7 mmol/L, five minutes after forced contraction), whereas ammonia rose from 14 to 489 μmol/L.

A skeletal muscle biopsy specimen was diagnostic for McArdle disease with subsarcolemmal vacuoles that contained glycogen (Figure 54.1). Myophosphorylase was absent in the muscle fibers. Biochemically, there was deficiency of the enzyme myophosphorylase (8 IU/L, normal >12–560 IU/L) in the muscle tissue. Sequencing of the gene revealed that she was compound heterozygote for two missense mutations on exons 4 and 12, respectively, of the PYGM (phosphorylase, glycogen, muscle) gene located on chromosome 11q13.

Follow-up

The patient was advised to avoid strenuous exercise. A carbohydrate-rich diet was prescribed. In subsequent years no weakness has developed.

Diagnostic considerations

The diagnosis of McArdle disease was considered on the basis of the clinical manifestations with exercise-induced cramps occurring after a few minutes and rapidly diminishing at rest, a normal neurological examination, and CK values >10 × ULN, in association with the marginal increase in serum lactate after exercise of the forearm muscles. Healthy persons may have mild CK elevation following exercise. The muscle biopsy showed vacuoles filled with glycogen and myophosphorylase staining was negative. DNA analysis ultimately proved the diagnosis.

General remarks

McArdle disease (glycogen storage disease type 5) is rare, but the most frequent of the carbohydrate metabolic myopathies. It was named after the British physician, Brian McArdle, who described the disease for the first time in 1951.

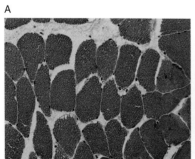 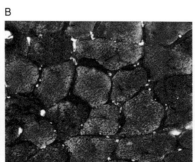 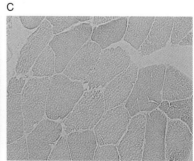

A   B   C

Figure 54.1. A skeletal muscle biopsy specimen showed small subsarcolemmal vacuoles on HE staining (A), and a positive periodic acid Schiff reaction, also at the subsarcolemmal level (B). The intense staining disappeared after digesting by diastase (not shown). A myophosphorylase staining showed no enzyme activity throughout the muscle fibers (C).

McArdle disease is caused by mutations in both alleles of the PYGM gene, which encodes for the myophosphorylase protein, the muscle isoform of glycogen phosphorylase. In most affected patients, there is no detectable glycogen phosphorylase activity. Because the liver and heart isoforms are produced normally, McArdle disease is a pure myopathy.

As one might expect in an autosomal recessive inherited disease, males and females are equally affected; there have been occasional reports of a carrier with a deficiency of muscle glycogen phosphorylase and muscle complaints.

The enzyme is involved in converting glycogen into glucose-1-phosphate. This, in turn, is converted to glucose-6-phosphate, which enters glycolysis and subsequently the Krebs cycle and oxidative phosphorylation to generate ATP under aerobic conditions. In patients with McArdle disease, glycolysis is blocked upstream, but patients can still absorb glucose from the blood and convert it into glucose-6-phosphate, which then enters the downstream steps of glycolysis.

Patients with McArdle disease suffer from exercise-related symptoms when brief and intense isometric muscle contractions take place, such as lifting a heavy object, or dynamic exercises with a high intensity, like climbing stairs or running. There is marked variation even within families. The onset can be in childhood but diagnosis is frequently delayed until after 30 years of age.

Initially, there is exercise-related fatigue, muscle stiffness, myalgia, and weakness, which is induced by exercise and relieved by rest. If exercise is sustained, contractures occur. One should ask whether the patient has experienced a "second wind" phenomenon, which is almost pathognomonic: a brief rest after myalgias allows further activity. Rhabdomyolysis is encountered in more than half of the patients after intense muscle contractions, and about 10% of these patients have renal failure, which is usually reversible but requires immediate treatment. Muscle weakness is usually mild and only seen in patients >40 years of age.

The diagnosis is based on the history and the inability of the patient to produce lactate during a forearm exercise test, lack of muscle glycogen phosphorylase activity on muscle biopsy and, more recently, DNA studies.

The ischemic lactate test, which was also performed in our patient, has been replaced recently by a nonischemic forearm test to avoid the potential risk of a compartment syndrome. The CK activity level can be very high with rhabdomyolysis, but is also elevated at rest in almost all patients. A recent Cochrane review showed that there was only low quality evidence of improvement in some parameters with creatine, oral sucrose, ramipril, and a carbohydrate-rich diet. It is, therefore, of utmost importance to educate the patient about the risks of rhabdomyolysis provoked by exercise as myoglobinuria may cause persistent renal insufficiency.

Rhabdomyolysis, acute muscle breakdown, is characterized by elevated creatine kinase activity ($>10 \times$ ULN; usually much higher), high serum concentrations of myoglobin, and possibly myoglobinuria (see Table 9). CK activity will decrease rapidly after a few days. Rhabdomyolysis can be accompanied by myalgia and weakness. Renal dysfunction and renal failure are the most severe complications of acute rhabdomyolysis. Rhabdomyolysis can have many causes. These include alcohol, drugs (cocaine, amphetamine), antipsychotic drugs and statins, infections, trauma, electrolyte disturbances, and hyperthermia. Neuromuscular disorders that can be associated with rhabdomyolysis are–among others–dystrophinopathy (Case 38), LGMD2I, (Case 41), malignant hyperthermia (Case 48), McArdle disease (present case), mitochondrial disease (Case 55), hypothyroidism, and rare hereditary disorders of metabolism. A systematic diagnostic work-up is needed to find the cause of rhabdomyolysis (Figure 54.2).

Suggested reading

David WS, Chad DA, Kambadakone A, Hedley-White ET. Case 7–2012: a 79-year-old man with pain and weakness in the legs. *New Engl J Med* 2012; **366**: 944–954.

Kazemi-Esfarjani P, Skomorowska E, Jensen TD, et al. A nonischemic forearm exercise test for McArdle disease. *Ann Neurol* 2002; **52**: 153–159.

Lucia A, Nogales-Gadea G, Pérez M, et al. McArdle's disease: what do neurologists need to know? *Nat Clin Pract Neurol* 2008; **4**: 568–577.

Quinlivan R, Martinuzzi A, Schoser B. Pharmacological and nutritional treatment for McArdle disease (Glycogen Storage Disease type V). *Cochrane Database Syst Rev* 2008; **2**: CD003458.

Quinlivan R, Buckley J, James M, et al. McArdle disease: a clinical review. *J Neurol Neurosurg Psychiatry* 2010; **81**: 1182–1188.

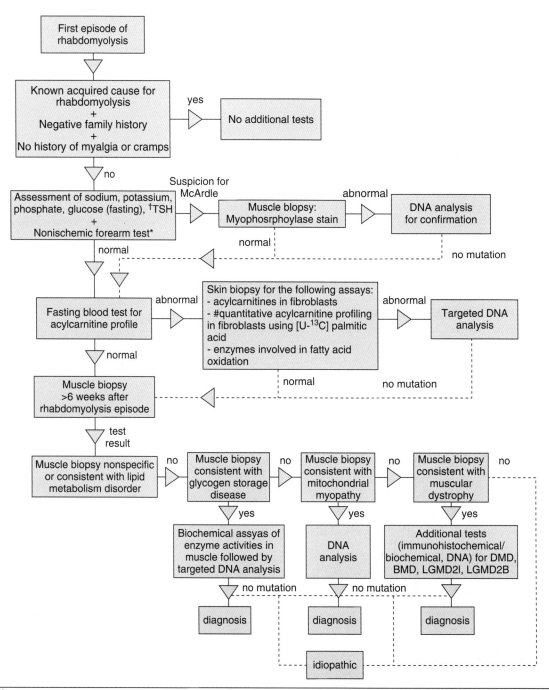

Diagnostic flowchart rhabdomyolysis

First episode of rhabdomyolysis

Known acquired cause for rhabdomyolysis + Negative family history + No history of myalgia or cramps

yes → No additional tests

no

Assessment of sodium, potassium, phosphate, glucose (fasting), †TSH + Nonischemic forearm test*

Suspicion for McArdle →

Muscle blopsy: Myophosrphoylase stain

abnormal → DNA analysis for confirmation

normal

no mutation

normal

Fasting blood test for acylcarnitine profile

abnormal → Skin biopsy for the following assays:
- acylcarnitines in fibroblasts
- #quantitative acylcarnitine profiling in fibroblasts using [U-^{13}C] palmitic acid
- enzymes involved in fatty acid oxidation

abnormal → Targeted DNA analysis

normal

normal

no mutation

Muscle biopsy >6 weeks after rhabdomyolysis episode

test result

Muscle biopsy nonspecific or consistent with lipid metabolism disorder

no → Muscle biopsy consistent with glycogen storage disease

no → Muscle biopsy consistent with mitochondrial myopathy

no → Muscle biopsy consistent with muscular dystrophy

no

yes

Biochemical assyas of enzyme activities in muscle followed by targeted DNA analysis

yes

DNA analysis

yes

Additional tests (immunohistochemical/ biochemical, DNA) for DMD, BMD, LGMD2I, LGMD2B

no mutation

no mutation

diagnosis

diagnosis

diagnosis

idiopathic

† TSH = Thyroid stimulating hormone * See Kazemi-Esfarjani P, et al., A Nonischemic forearm exercise test for McArdle disease. *Ann Neurol* 2002; **52**: 153-159, # A method for the investigation of mitochondrial fatty acid beta-oxldation in cultured fibroblasts. Monolayer cultures are incubated with palmitic acid and L-carnitine and the acylcarnitines produced by the cells are extracted from the cell suspension and analyzed. DMD = Duchenne muscular dystrophy; BMD = Becker muscular dystrophy; LGMD = limb girdle muscular dystrophy.

Figure 54.2. A flowchart for the diagnostic work-up of a patient with rhabdomyolysis.

Mitochondrial disease: progressive external ophthalmoplegia: a woman with drooping eyelids

Clinical history

This 52-year-old woman visited the neurologist because of drooping eyelids, which had not changed much over the past ten years. Old photographs showed slight drooping from her mid-teens onward. At one point, she had experienced transient double vision. Speaking, swallowing, and muscle strength were normal.

Examination

There was symmetric ptosis partly covering the pupils when looking straight ahead, which was not worse when looking upward or laterally. Eye movements were intact and there was no diplopia.

Ancillary investigations

Single fiber EMG was normal, excluding a neuromuscular transmission deficit. A muscle biopsy taken from the deltoid muscle confirmed a diagnosis of mitochondrial myopathy (Figure 55.1). Subsequently, DNA analysis of leukocytes revealed the presence of the recessive pathogenic p.A467T and [p.T251I;p.P587L]

mutations in the POLG1 gene, which explains the clinical phenotype.

Diagnostic considerations

Arguments against classic myasthenia gravis (Case 34) were:

- Slow and steady progression
- Symmetric ptosis
- Absence of evident diplopia
- No worsening on looking upward or sideways (see Table 34.1)

Arguments against myotonic dystrophy type 1 (Case 50) were:

- Absence of myotonia and distal muscle atrophy
- Negative family history

Arguments against OPMD (Case 46) were:

- Absence of dysphagia
- Negative family history

A mitochondrial disease was a likely alternative explanation. In patients with this typical mitochondrial

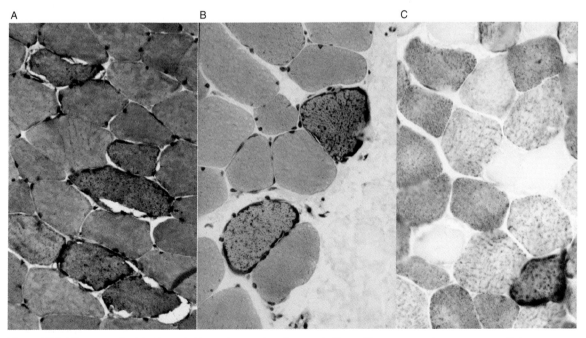

A   B   C

Figure 55.1. HE staining of a deltoid muscle biopsy shows at least five muscle fibers with a more granular appearance and intense subsarcolemmal staining (A). The fibers appear somewhat distorted. With the modified Gomori trichrome staining (B), the abnormal fibers are even more obvious and two "ragged-red" muscle fibers can be observed. The mitochondrial cytochrome oxidase staining shows both fibers without staining and abnormal subsarcolemmal staining suggesting accumulation, usually abnormal, of mitochondria (C).

presentation of chronic progressive external ophthalmoplegia (CPEO), it is currently justified to refrain from performing a skeletal muscle biopsy and to start the diagnostic process with analysis of the POLG1 gene in a blood sample.

Follow-up

Ten years after presentation, this patient reported no change in symptoms.

General remarks

Mitochondrial respiratory chain dysfunction results in defective ATP generation and can present at any age, potentially affecting any organ. In adults, mitochondrial disease usually manifests as a neuromuscular disorder or CNS disorder (Tables 55.1 and 55.2).

Hereditary mitochondrial diseases can be caused by mutations in the mitochondrial or nuclear DNA. Many adult mitochondrial phenotypes, including CPEO can be caused by mutations in the mitochondrial DNA (mtDNA). The genes involved encode components of the respiratory chain, or as in CPEO, tRNA molecules necessary for intramitochondrial protein synthesis. Defects in mitochondrial DNA are usually maternally inherited. Exceptions are deletions that, in general, are sporadic.

Most information for the formation and maintenance of the individual subunits of the respiratory chain is encoded by nuclear genes. Diseases that result from these mutations have a Mendelian inheritance. Nuclear genes also encode enzymes necessary for the constant replication of mitochondrial (mt)DNA. Mutations in these nuclear genes thus cause secondary mtDNA defects, often multiple deletions or depletion resulting in a reduction in the amount of mtDNA. AD and AR CPEO can be caused by mutations in several nuclear genes involved in mtDNA replication, the most important of which is the gene for the catalytic subunit of polymerase gamma (POLG). Mutations in other nuclear genes affecting mtDNA integrity, all causing AD CPEO, include: POLG2, encoding the accessory subunit of POLG; SLC25A4, encoding adenine nucleotide translocator 1; and the PEO1 gene, encoding the mitochondrial Twinkle helicase (Figure 55.2).

POLG mutations in particular can result in extremely heterogeneous phenotypes. Especially in infancy and childhood, a POLG mutation can cause Alpers syndrome (psychomotor retardation, epilepsy, and liver failure) or Alpers-like syndromes with proximal myopathy or hypotonia. Sodium valproate given for seizure control can trigger liver failure in patients with a POLG mitochondrial disease.

In adolescence and adulthood, CPEO can occur as an isolated or part of a more complex syndrome such as large fiber sensory neuropathy (SANDO) (see Table 7). Other POLG-related features are proximal myopathy, parkinsonism, cerebellar ataxia, myoclonus, various forms of epilepsy, diabetes mellitus, and early menopause. Increasingly, previously healthy young adults are diagnosed with progressive epilepsy and

Table 55.1. Common features of mitochondrial disease

- Muscle weakness and exercise intolerance
- CPEO (see Introduction, Figure 11)
- Cardiomyopathy (see Table 38.1)
- Sensorineural hearing loss
- Ataxia
- Peripheral neuropathy
- Diabetes
- Myoclonus and epilepsy
- Retinitis pigmentosa
- Leukoencephalopathy on brain imaging

Frequently these features occur in combination. Fatigue is a rather nonspecific feature of mitochondrial disease. Rhabdomyolysis has been observed.

Table 55.2. Mitochondrial syndromes with prominent or predominant neuromuscular signs in adults

- CPEO
- Kearns–Sayre syndrome (KSS): onset <20 years, CPEO, retinitis pigmentosa plus one of the following features: ataxia, cardiac conduction block, CSF protein >1 g/L
- Mitochondrial encephalomyopathy with lactic acidosis and stroke-like episodes (MELAS)
- Myoclonus epilepsy with ragged red fibers (MERRF)
- Mitochondrial neurogastrointestinal encephalomyopathy (MNGIE): gastrointestinal dysmotility, cachexia, CPEO, peripheral neuropathy, and leukoencephalopathy
- Neuropathy, ataxia, and retinitis pigmentosa (NARP)
- Sensory ataxic neuropathy with ophthalmoplegia, dysarthria, and ophthalmoplegia (SANDO) syndrome

Identical mutations in mitochondrial genes may cause protean phenotypic features; similar phenotypes can be caused by different mutations. As more patients with hereditary mitochondrial cytopathies are being recognized, the variation of phenotypes will increase.

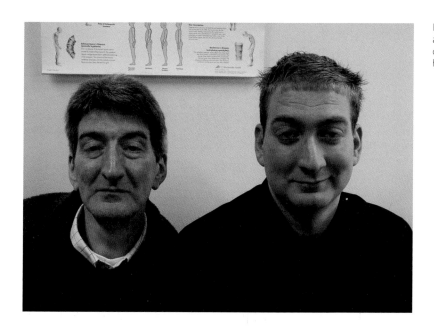

Figure 55.2. Father and son with ptosis and progressive external ophthalmoplegia caused by a mitochondrial Twinkle helicase mutation.

epileptic visual aura as the first manifestation of a POLG mutation. The present case has a mild phenotype and forms another part of the spectrum.

At present, a diagnosis of CPEO, caused by a POLG mutation (or a mutation in another nuclear gene), can be reached relatively easily by investigating DNA extracted from blood. The detection of primary mtDNA defects may be more difficult because the amount of mutated mtDNA may be too low in the blood (examination of urine may have a higher yield) and sometimes decreases with age. If the clinical syndrome suggests mitochondrial disease, but genetic examination of blood and urine for common mutations in mtDNA and nuclear DNA is negative, a muscle biopsy should be performed to confirm mitochondrial abnormalities (ragged red fibers, cytochrome c oxidase-negative fibers). This can be followed by various molecular genetic techniques to detect mtDNA abnormalities and by biochemical analyses of respiratory chain activities.

Management of CPEO includes advice on the symptomatic treatment of ptosis leading to functional blindness and social handicap. Ptosis may be alleviated by prosthetic inserts placed inside spectacles to raise the eyelids. Some patients prefer surgical correction. Symptomatic treatment of other mitochondrial symptoms should be offered accordingly. Pharmacological treatment options directed at the biochemical defect are limited. High-dose coenzyme Q_{10} could be

beneficial only if coenzyme Q_{10}, a mobile electron carrier in the mitochondrial inner membrane, is deficient. Genetic advice in case of a POLG or other nuclear gene mutation follows the Mendelian rules. In the case of an mtDNA defect, it is more difficult to provide accurate genetic counseling.

Suggested reading

Blok MJ, van den Bosch BJ, Jongen E, et al. The unfolding clinical spectrum of POLG mutations. *J Med Genet* 2009; **46**: 776–785.

Koopman WJ, Willems PH, Smeitink JA. Monogenic mitochondrial disorders. *New Engl J Med* 2012; **366**: 1132–1141.

McFarland R, Taylor RW, Turnbull DM. A neurological perspective on mitochondrial disease. *Lancet Neurol* 2010; **9**: 829–840.

Rahman S, Hanna MG. Diagnosis and therapy in neuromuscular disorders: diagnosis and new treatments in mitochondrial diseases. *J Neurol Neurosurg Psychiatry* 2009; **80**: 943–953.

Tang S, Dimberg EL, Milone M, Wong LJ. Mitochondrial neurogastrointestinal encephalomyelopathy (MNGIE)-like phenotype: an expanded clinical spectrum of POLG1 mutations. *J Neurol* 2012; **259**: 862–868.

Visser N, Braun KP, Van den Bergh WM, et al. Juvenile-onset Alpers syndrome: interpreting MRI findings. *Neurology* 2010; **74**: 1231–1233.

Myositis: a woman with subacute, progressive weakness and high creatine kinase

Clinical history

This 33-year-old, previously healthy woman noticed exercise-induced muscle and joint pain, and discoloration of her fingers. A few months later, she also experienced progressive fatigue. Shortly thereafter she noticed difficulty lifting her arms and climbing stairs and she had a problem swallowing. Muscle weakness increased over a period of months, and at an accelerated rate during the week prior to presentation.

Examination

The findings on presentation were a dropped head, bulbar dysarthria, difficulty swallowing, and weakness of the deltoid muscles (MRC 3), biceps brachii muscles (MRC 4), iliopsoas muscles (MRC 3), and other proximal leg muscles (MRC 4). There were no skin abnormalities.

Ancillary investigations

Serum CK activity was 2520 U/L (17 × ULN), increasing to 3735 U/L in one week. The MRI scan showed edema in various muscles and hematoxylin and eosin (HE) staining of a deltoid muscle biopsy showed perimysial and perivascular mononuclear cell infiltrates and necrotic and regenerative muscle fibers (Figure 56.1). Myositis-specific autoantibodies were absent.

Diagnostic considerations

The rapidly progressive symmetric muscle weakness, the absence of skin abnormalities, and the rising levels of CK prompted a diagnosis of polymyositis, which was confirmed by muscle biopsy.

Follow-up

The patient was admitted and placed on high-dose corticosteroids (1–1.5 mg/kg/d). After initial further deterioration in muscle strength, CK levels began to decrease after two weeks, followed by a gradual increase in muscle strength during the following two weeks. Prednisolone was tapered very slowly after six weeks, and four years after onset, she had normal muscle strength and normal CK on a maintenance low-dose prednisolone regimen. Adverse effects of treatment were hypertension and weight gain. The rheumatologist diagnosed an unspecified connective tissue disease. She could not resume her job as a secretary because of persistent fatigue.

General remarks

The clinical hallmark of the autoimmune idiopathic inflammatory myopathies (with the exception of sporadic inclusion body myositis (IBM), Case 57) is subacute progression during weeks to months of proximal weakness, notably of the deltoid and

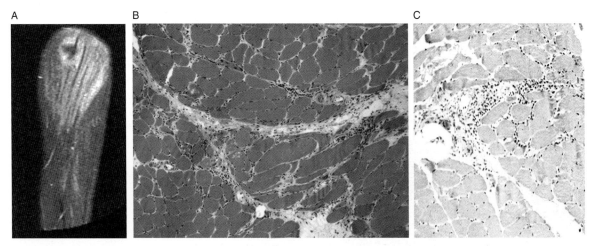

Figure 56.1. T2-STIR MRI of the right upper arms shows edema of the deltoid muscle (A). HE staining of the muscle biopsy shows variation of fiber size, perifascicular atrophy of muscle fibers, perimysial and endomysial inflammatory infiltrates in the fascicles and around blood vessels, and necrosis of muscle fibers (B); and perivascular infiltrate (C).

iliopsoas muscles. Distal weakness, dysphagia, and respiratory insufficiency may evolve during the course of the disease, if untreated. Several types of myositis have been differentiated, based on clinical and histopathological features.

Dermatomyositis is associated with typical skin abnormalities (Table 56.1; Figure 56.2). CK activity is elevated in most patients, but the diagnosis should not be discarded if the CK activity is normal. The muscle biopsy shows perivascular, perimysial mononuclear cells, primarily macrophages, B-cells, and CD4+ cells. The characteristic perifascicular atrophy is found in less than half of adult patients with dermatomyositis, and is often absent early in the disease. According to current guidelines, it is not mandatory to perform a muscle biopsy if the clinical presentation includes the typical skin changes of dermatomyositis. Dermatomyositis is associated with malignancies and with systemic lupus erythematosus.

Polymyositis is a much used, but confusing term. Initially, it was applied to patients with subacute proximal weakness without skin abnormalities, and with inflammation of muscle tissue without perifascicular atrophy, sometimes in combination with an autoimmune connective tissue disease (overlap syndromes). Later, the definition of polymyositis was based exclusively on a specific histopathological feature: in addition to perimysial infiltrates, the diagnosis now required the presence of endomysial localized inflammatory infiltrates consisting of cytotoxic T-cells, which invade non-necrotic muscle fibers. This feature is also specifically found in IBM. Most, if not all patients diagnosed with polymyositis on the basis of this pathological finding, turned out to have IBM, and did not respond to immunosupressant treatment. Recently, it has been suggested that the term polymyositis be used for patients with nonspecific perimysial and endomysial localizations of inflammation, not requiring invasion of nonnecrotic muscle fibers for the diagnosis. Defined in this way,

Table 56.1. Characteristic dermatological abnormalities in dermatomyositis

- Heliotrope (purplish) periorbital edema
- Raised erythematous lesions over the knuckles, elbows, knees, medial malleoli (Gottron sign)
- Erythematous, sometimes macular, rash over the extensor surfaces of the elbows and knees, in the face, neck and anterior chest (V-sign), and back of the neck (shawl sign)
- Periungual telangiectasia

Subcutaneous calcifications occur in juvenile dermatomyositis, but not in adults.

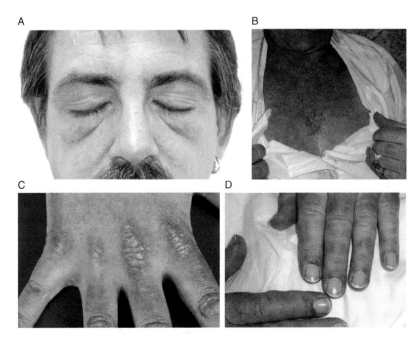

A   B

C   D

Figure 56.2. Skin changes in dermatomyositis: periorbital edema with a reddish-purplish (heliotrope) discoloration (A); scaly rash of the upper chest (B); scaly, slightly elevated rash of the knuckles and dorsal surface of the fingers (Gottron's sign or papules, C); periungual erythematic and capillary changes (D).

most patients with myositis will be classified as having polymyositis, with or without an associated connective tissue disease. If there is invasion of non-necrotic muscle fibers, sporadic IBM is the most likely diagnosis (Case 57).

In some patients with a clinical presentation of myositis (subacute onset and progression over weeks or months; proximal weakness) and good response to high-dose corticosteroids, the muscle biopsy reveals necrotic and regenerating fibers, but no or little cell infiltration (immune-mediated necrotizing myopathy). It is important to differentiate this condition from muscular dystrophies, especially as the weakness may be severe and CK may be strongly elevated. In case of diagnostic doubt, the doctor may be tempted to underdose and shorten a therapeutic "trial" with prednisone, which will lead to a false diagnosis of muscular dystrophy if the patient seems not to respond. The immune-mediated necrotizing myopathy condition is associated with malignancies.

Other types of inflammatory myopathies include granulomatous myositis and eosinophilic myofascitis. Infectious agents are rarely involved. In many muscular dystrophies, mononuclear infiltrates can be found in a muscle biopsy specimen.

The treatment of myositis consists of high-dose corticosteroids (in the case of prednisone, 1–1.5 mg/kg/d for at least four weeks followed by slow tapering). Undertreatment, which may follow from the wish to minimalize adverse effects, is the most important reason for treatment failure. Treatment with IVIg has been shown to be beneficial in a short-duration RCT, and can be considered in case of life-threatening situations such as severe bulbar weakness. Other treatments, such as methotrexate, azathioprine, ciclosporin A, eculizumab, infliximab, and etanercept yielded negative results in RCTs and were associated with significant side effects. Yet, these may be considered as second-line therapies.

The long-term outcome of myositis is disappointing. Only a small minority of patients regain normal quality of life without medication. Almost half the patients with favorable clinical outcome remain dependent on medication, especially patients with anti-Jo-1 autoantibodies, concomitant interstitial lung disease, and arthritis (anti-synthetase syndrome). Cancer and lung complications are the main causes of disease-related mortality in about 10% of cases.

Use of statins can cause elevated CK activity and even rhabdomyolysis. In most patients, CK activity returns to normal values following cessation of statins. Some patients develop immune-mediated necrotizing myopathy that is characterized by proximal muscle weakness during the use of statins, CK elevation, and persistence of weakness and of elevated CK activity despite discontinuation of statins. The muscle biopsy shows signs of necrotizing myopathy without inflammation. Immunosuppressive drugs can be effective.

Suggested reading

Amato AA, Barohn RJ. Evaluation and treatment of inflammatory myopathies. *J Neurol Neurosurg Psychiatry* 2009; **80**: 1060–1068.

Bronner IM, van der Meulen MF, de Visser M, et al. Long-term outcome in polymyositis and dermatomyositis. *Ann Rheum Dis* 2006; **65**: 1456–1461.

Gordon P, Winer JB, Hoogendijk JE, Choy EH. Immunosuppressant and immunomodulatory treatment for dermatomyositis and polymyositis. *Cochrane Database Syst Rev* 2012; **8**: CD003463.

Grable-Esposito P, Katzberg HD, Greenberg SA, et al. Immune-mediated necrotizing myopathy associated with statins. *Muscle Nerve* 2010; **41**: 185–190.

Mastaglia FL. Inflammatory muscle diseases. *Neurol India* 2008; **56**: 263–270.

Zong M, Lundberg IE. Pathogenesis, classification and treatment of inflammatory myopathies. *Nat Rev Rheumatol* 2011; **7**: 297–306.

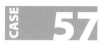

Sporadic inclusion body myositis: an 81-year-old woman with a tendency to fall

Clinical history

The patient, a retired nurse and grandmother, had always been very active. She liked to make long-distance walks. From the age of 77 years, she increasingly experienced frequent and unexpected falls. Subsequently, she noticed progressive difficulty with walking, which stimulated her to use a rollator. If she reached for an object on a shelf she had to support her arm. Recently, she noticed difficulty swallowing. She sometimes choked on food.

Examination

On inspection, no abnormalities of the facial muscles were found. Oculomotor function was normal. The tongue was not atrophic and movements were undisturbed. She had overt atrophy of the thigh muscles. Fasciculation was absent. Manual muscle testing demonstrated more or less symmetric, mild to moderate weakness (MRC grade 4–5 to 4) of the neck flexors, deltoid and upper arm muscles, deep finger flexors, interosseus muscles, and iliopsoas muscles. The quadriceps femoris muscles showed severe weakness (MRC grade 3). The myotatic reflexes were reduced.

Ancillary investigations

Serum CK activity was slightly elevated (2 × ULN). CT scans of the thigh muscles showed severely wasted quadriceps femoris muscles, which were virtually replaced by fatty tissue (Figure 57.1).

A muscle biopsy taken from a triceps brachii muscle showed marked variation in the size of the muscle fibers, signs of degeneration and regeneration, numerous muscle fibers with rimmed vacuoles and prominent cell infiltrates located in the endomysium, consisting of CD8-positive T-lymphocytes and, to a lesser extent, CD4+ T-lymphocytes and macrophages. There were numerous cytochrome oxidase negative muscle fibers and ragged red fibers (Figure 57.2).

Diagnostic considerations

Based on the deep finger flexor muscle weakness, the severe CT abnormalities of the quadriceps femoris muscle, and the pathological abnormalities, the diagnosis of sporadic inclusion body myositis (sIBM) could be made.

Follow-up

No immunosuppressive or immunomodulative treatment was given. She had gradual decline but remained ambulatory.

General remarks

sIBM is a degenerative muscle disease albeit with prominent inflammation, which is treatment-resistant. sIBM runs a slowly progressive course. Rimmed vacuoles and inclusions, which contain ectopic proteins, are present within IBM muscle fibers. Inflammation accumulates primarily at endomysial sites, where predominantly CD8+ T-cells and macrophages but also some B-cells, plasma cells, and dendritic cells actively invade non-necrotic muscle fibers.

sIBM usually manifests at the end of the sixth decade of life and rarely around the age of 40 years.

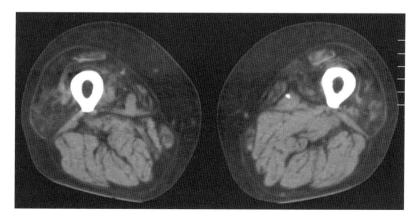

Figure 57.1. CT scan through the middle of the thigh shows atrophy and replacement by fat of the quadriceps femoris, sartorius, and gracilis muscles with relative preservation of the biceps femoris, semitendinosus, and semimembranosus muscles.

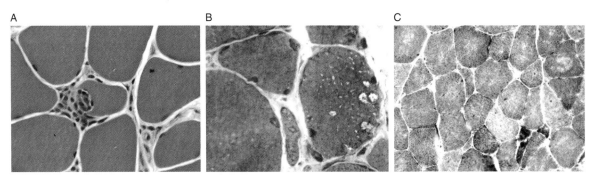

Figure 57.2. Triceps brachii muscle biopsy. The HE staining shows a collection of lymphocytes that are located in the endomysium and infiltrating a nonnecrotic muscle fiber (A). The modified Gomori trichrome staining shows a muscle fiber with the so-called rimmed vacuoles (B). Numerous cytochrome oxidase-negative muscle fibers can be observed (C).

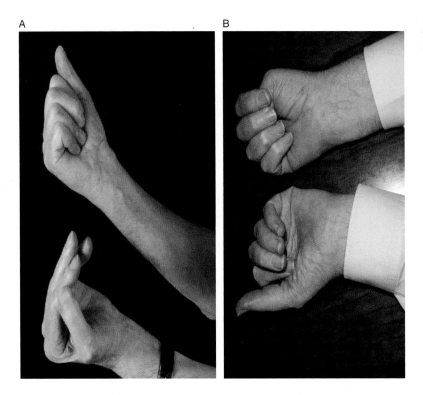

Figure 57.3. Weakness of the deep finger flexor muscles of the left hand in two patients with sporadic IBM (A, B).

Males are more frequently affected. The prevalence of sporadic IBM is variable in different populations and ethnic groups. The prevalence may range from 4.9 per million inhabitants of the Netherlands to 10.7 per million in Connecticut, USA, and even 14.9 per million inhabitants of Western Australia. In 2000, survey prevalence was 51.3 per million in persons over 50 years of age.

Onset is most frequent in the quadriceps femoris and less common in the deep finger flexor muscles (Figure 57.3) and pharyngeal muscles.

sIBM affects both proximal and distal muscles, the ventrally located muscles being affected more than the dorsal. Weakness is slowly progressive, and often asymmetric. Neck extensors ("dropped head"), shoulder and hip abductors, and abductor and opponens pollicis muscles are relatively spared, allowing some grip function of the hands. Facial weakness is observed in 40% of the cases. It can be severe and it may cause inability to close the eyes, especially in females. Neither myalgia nor muscle cramps are a feature of IBM.

In sIBM, sCK is <5 times the normal value in 80% of patients; 10% may have CK values >10 × ULN.

sIBM is a mimic of the LMN variant of ALS. EMG is not always helpful in distinguishing sIBM from ALS, as neurogenic MUPs can also be found in sIBM. A skeletal muscle biopsy can help to make the distinction. Diagnostic criteria for IBM, proposed in 1995, strongly emphasize histopathological features. It has recently been stressed, however, that in patients with the clinical features of IBM, the diagnosis should not be rejected if these histopathological abnormalities, like rimmed vacuoles or amyloid deposits, are absent. There is, as yet, no consensus on whether the diagnosis can be established on the basis of the clinical picture only.

IBM was believed to be a rather mild disorder. A recent study has shown that sIBM is a disabling disorder albeit with normal life expectancy. Patients become wheelchair-dependent approximately 15 years after onset of the disease, and cachexia is a frequent finding. Cause of death is usually pneumonia, which may be attributed to aspiration from the associated dysphagia. All immunosuppresive treatment strategies that have been proven to be more or less successful in other idiopathic inflammatory myopathies, like dermatomyositis and myositis associated with connective tissue disease, unfortunately have failed in sIBM. Supportive strategies may improve quality of life. The effect of noninvasive respiratory support has yet to be established. In patients with severe dysphagia in whom dietary measures are insufficient, cricopharyngeotomy can be considered (see Case 46).

Suggested reading

Cox FM, Titulaer MJ, Sont JK, et al. A 12-year follow-up in sporadic inclusion body myositis: an end stage with major disabilities. *Brain* 2011; **134**: 3167–3175.

Benveniste O, Guiguet M, Freebody J, et al. Long-term observational study of sporadic inclusion body myositis. *Brain* 2011; **134**: 3176–3184.

Benveniste O, Hilton-Jones D. Workshop report. International workshop on inclusion body myositis held at the Institute of Myology, Paris, on 29 May 2009. *Neuromusc Disord* 2012; **20**: 414–421.

Greenberg SA. Inclusion body myositis: review of recent literature. *Curr Neurol Neurosci Rep* 2009; **9**: 83–89.

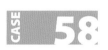

CASE 58 Sarcoid myopathy: a church-goer who could no longer attend Sunday vespers

Clinical history

For the previous six months, this 40-year-old woman had experienced a gradual increase in difficulty in walking. She lived in a low-care home. For two years, the walking difficulties had been noticed by her mother. They used to walk together to church, twice on Sundays, and she continued to attend the morning service, albeit with great effort and pain. When seated she prayed and sang with tears in her eyes because of increasing pain in the lower back, pelvis, and upper legs. Climbing stairs had become almost impossible. She had visited a specialist in rehabilitation medicine who had advised installing a stairlift.

Examination

She was slightly short of breath. Muscle strength of the arms was normal, but the biceps brachii tendon reflex was negative. When standing and walking, she had to position the upper half of her body backward in order to remain in an upright position. When rising from a chair, she had to bend the upper half of her body forward. Both phenomena suggest weakness of the lower erector trunci and hip flexion muscles. Scoliosis was absent.

She had atrophy of the muscles of the upper legs but normal calves. We found a limb girdle pattern of weakness of the legs with normal strength of the quadriceps femoris muscles. Weakness of the adductor muscles was MRC grade 4 in the left and 3 in the right leg.

Sensation was normal. The Achilles tendon reflexes were negative. She had pes equinus suggesting chronic weakness of the foot extensor muscles.

Ancillary investigations

The referring neurologist found slight CK elevation of 1.5 × ULN. A spinal tap showed no pleocytosis and a

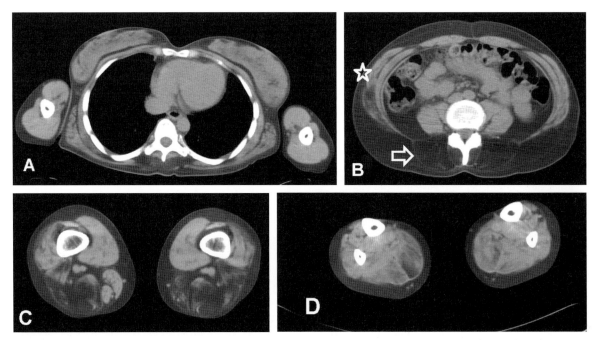

Figure 58.1. CT scans show abnormal erector trunci muscles at the thoracic (A), and lumbosacral levels (B, arrow), and also abnormal abdominal wall muscles (asterisk). (C) Abnormal lateral vastus muscles with marked replacement by fat of the biceps femoris, semitendinosus, and semimembranosus muscles. The foot extensor muscles are atrophic (D).

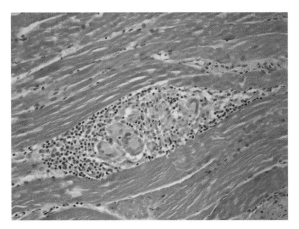

Figure 58.2. A medial vastus muscle biopsy (hematoxylin-and-eosin staining) shows a nonnecrotizing granulomatous inflammatory lesion and several multinucleate giant cells, confirming a diagnosis of sarcoid myopathy.

normal protein level. Oligoclonal IgG bands and a high IgG-index of 0.93 suggested intrathecal immunoglobulin synthesis. Somatosensory responses after stimulation of the tibial nerves were negative. The MRI scan of the head showed two small periventricular hyperintense lesions; the spinal MRI was normal.

We found a low forced VC of 62%. EMG abnormalities were compatible with coexisting myopathy and sensory neuropathy. A CT scan showed severe abnormalities in clinically affected and nonaffected muscles (Figure 58.1). A biopsy of the medial vastus muscle showed mild neurogenic abnormalities, but also prominent inflammatory abnormalities with giant cells suggesting sarcoidosis (Figure 58.2). A chest radiograph showed mild interstitial pneumonitis but no hilar lymphadenopathy. The serum ACE concentration was increased. An internist performed a lymph node biopsy that confirmed the diagnosis of sarcoidosis.

Diagnostic considerations

The patient experienced progressive walking difficulties over a period of months caused by weakness of the pelvic girdle and leg muscles, and pain and mild sensory neuropathy. The combination of myopathic and neurogenic abnormalities with progression over months excludes one of the limb girdle muscular dystrophies, Pompe disease, and IBM. Myositis in combination with an autoimmune connective tissue disease (Case 56) can be associated with neuropathy. In order to differentiate, a muscle biopsy is indicated.

Table 58.1. Neuromuscular manifestations of neurosarcoidosis

- Peripheral neuropathy (frequent): solitary or multiple neuropathies, polyradiculopathy, and non-length dependent sensory or sensorimotor neuropathy. Positive neuropathic features and pain are prominent features. Damaged nerves can be vulnerable to compression

- Polyradiculoneuropathy (rare) can be rapidly progressive, or chronic progressive (atypical CIDP)

- Small-fiber neuropathy: distal pain is the hallmark. Autonomic symptoms form part of the clinical spectrum

- Solitary granulomatous muscle lesions are a frequent and usually asymptomatic finding. Palpable nodular lesions are rare

- Acute or chronic more extensive inflammatory myopathy

Follow-up

The patient had a combination of peripheral neuropathy and inflammatory myopathy.

She was treated with steroids, which improved her walking distance. After a follow-up of five years on low-dose steroids, she could still walk using a rollator.

General remarks

Sarcoidosis is a systemic inflammatory multisystem disorder that is characterized by noncaseating granulomatous inflammation. It is probably a multifactorial disease involving genetic and microbial factors. Genes in the main histocompatibility complex region play a dominant role. Immunological hallmarks include expression of cytokines, including IL-2, that are produced by type 1 T-helper cells, and tumor necrosis factor at the site of inflammation. Myeloid dendritic cells probably play a role as antigen-presenting cells. Candidate microbial triggers include mycobacteria and propionibacteria. There are no clinically useful biomarkers.

The lungs, intrathoracic lymph nodes, skin, and eyes are most commonly affected. Sarcoidosis can implicate any part of the nervous system and any muscle. Up to 5% of patients with sarcoidosis have clinical signs of neurosarcoidosis and most actually present with neurosarcoidosis.

Neurosarcoidosis may manifest as an acute neurological syndrome resulting from a cerebral mass lesion, or aseptic meningitis. Involvement of the basal meninges may cause cranial neuritis. Cranial neuropathy can also result from isolated nerve granulomas, or increased intracranial pressure. Unilateral or bilateral facial nerve palsies are most frequent.

Spinal sarcoidosis can occur at any level. Intramedullary lesions may lead to a chronic myelopathy syndrome. Cauda equina neurosarcoidosis is characterized by thickened nerve roots with leptomeningeal contrast enhancement.

Neuromuscular manifestations of sarcoidosis, on the whole, are due to two causes, the first being nerve lesions resulting from inflammation with or without evidence of noncaseinating epitheloid granulomas (Table 58.1). The second cause, less well defined, leads to more generalized neuropathy probably as a result of inflammatory agents.

The diagnosis of neurosarcoidosis can be difficult and time-consuming if systemic manifestations are absent. Serum ACE levels are frequently normal. EMG can help to discriminate between axonal and demyelinating neuropathy. Axonal degeneration is far more prominent than demyelination. CT and MRI can help to localize lesions. A sensory nerve biopsy can reveal epineural or perineural granulomas and a skeletal muscle biopsy can show characteristic granulomas thereby confirming a diagnosis of sarcoidosis in patients with neuropathy.

Treatment consists of oral corticosteroids for months or even years, but unfortunately, not all patients respond. There is no evidence for efficacy of other immunosuppressive or immunomodulatory treatment strategies with the exception of a combination of mycophenolate mofetil and infliximab, or monotherapy with infliximab.

Suggested reading

Burns TM, Dyck PJ, Aksamit AJ, Dyck PJ. The natural history and long-term outcome of 57 limb sarcoidosis neuropathy cases. *J Neurol Sci* 2006; **15**: 77–87.

Chen ES, Moller DR. Sarcoidosis–scientific progress and clinical challenges. *Nat Rev Rheumatol* 2011; **12**: 457–467.

Hoitsma E, Faber CG, Drent M, Sharma OP. Neurosarcoidosis: a clinical dilemma. *Lancet Neurol* 2004; **3**: 397–407.

Reda H, Taylor SW, Klein CJ, Boes CJ. A case of sensory ataxia as the presenting manifestation of neurosarcoidosis. *Muscle Nerve* 2011; **43**: 900–905.

Tateyama M, Fujihara K, Itoyama Y. Dendritic cells in muscle lesions of sarcoidosis. *Hum Pathol* 2011; **42**: 340–346.

Vital A, Lagueny A, Ferrer X, et al. Sarcoid neuropathy: clinico-pathological study of 4 new cases and review of the literature. *Clin Neuropathol* 2008; **27**: 96–105.

Hypothyroid myopathy: a man with hypothyroidism erroneously diagnosed as muscular dystrophy

Clinical history

A 41-year-old male was referred with a six-month history of progressive, exercise-related muscle pains, cramps, and muscle weakness. His past medical history was unremarkable, and the family history was negative for neuromuscular disorders.

Examination

He had slight wasting and weakness of his shoulder girdle muscles. We also noted increased lumbar lordosis, firm calves, and a positive Gowers' phenomenon. Sensation and reflexes were normal.

Ancillary investigations

Serum CK activity was 3530 IU/L (N <130 IU/L). GAA activity in leukocytes was normal.

A biopsy from the quadriceps femoris muscle showed marked variation in the size of the muscle fibers, necrotic and regenerating fibers, areas of decreased oxidative enzyme activity in numerous muscle fibers, and subsarcolemmal accumulations of glycogen (Figure 59.1).

Immunohistochemical analysis, including dystrophin and sarcoglycan stains, was normal.

DNA analysis for mutations in the dystrophin gene (BMD, Case 38) and in chromosome 4q35 (FSHD, Case 43) was negative.

Diagnostic considerations

The progressive muscle weakness with a limb girdle distribution and markedly elevated serum CK could be consistent with muscular dystrophy and Pompe's

disease, despite the seemingly subacute onset and progression over months. During the work-up, however, the patient's condition deteriorated progressively. Muscle weakness increased. He developed nasal dysarthria, and sleep-apnea syndrome. The work-up of the latter includes analysis of thyroid gland function. The patient was found to have markedly increased TSH (185 mE/L, normal 0.4–4 mE/L). Free T4 was considerably decreased <2 mE/L (normal 10–23 mE/L), and anti-thyroid peroxidase antibodies were present. These findings led to a diagnosis of autoimmune thyroiditis manifesting with hypothyroidism and myopathy.

Follow-up

With treatment for hypothyroidism he had complete recovery. All symptoms and signs subsided.

General remarks

The endocrinological history of hypothyroidism includes tiredness, dry skin, cold intolerance, coarse voice, increase in weight, swelling of the tongue, and periorbital puffiness.

A prospective cohort study of newly diagnosed patients with hypothyroidism in a general hospital and a case–control study showed that neuromuscular symptoms were present in most patients with untreated primary hypothyroidism. Muscle complaints included weakness (54%), and fatigability, muscle pain, stiffness or cramps (42%). Few patients had muscle complaints as the presenting symptom. Distal sensory symptoms occurred in 29%.

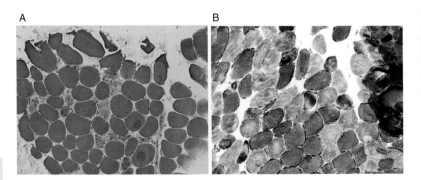

Figure 59.1. A biopsy from the quadriceps femoris muscle showed marked variation in the size of the muscle fibers, necrotic and regenerating fibers (HE stain) (A), and areas of decreased oxidative enzyme activity in numerous muscle fibers (NADH-TR stain) (B).

Detectable proximal muscle weakness was found in 30%–40%. Weakness was mild, MRC grade 4–5. Neck flexor, deltoid, and iliopsoas muscles were affected predominantly. About a third of patients had – usually bilateral – carpal tunnel syndrome. Mild, predominantly sensory axonal neuropathy is less frequent. In addition, one-third of patients had myopathic EMG abnormalities with short duration motor unit action potentials. Diagnostic delay ranged between two months and seven years (mean one year).

During treatment, muscle complaints resolved in 79% of the patients with an average time of seven months. Some patients remained symptomatic after one year of treatment. A significant correlation between the level of weakness and the biochemical severity of hypothyroidism in hypothyroid patients was not found. A mild myopathy is a likely explanation. Only in a few cases was myxedema or rhabdomyolysis observed. Muscle weakness preceding hypothyroidism is rare.

Serum CK is usually elevated, and sometimes strikingly high. Muscle biopsy may present nonspecific findings: rarely necrotic fibers and cell infiltrates, and core-like structures.

The main message of this case vignette is that all patients who present with an elevated CK could benefit from routine testing of serum TSH.

To illustrate this further, hyperthyroidism can be associated with neuromuscular symptoms such as weakness, fatigability, muscle pain, and cramps. On examination, mild weakness can be found. The EMG and CK activity is normal in most hyperthyroid patients with neuromuscular symptoms, and recovery following treatment is rapid. A functional muscle disorder is a more likely explanation than myopathy. Rarely, rhabdomyolysis may be associated with hyperthyroidism.

Suggested reading

Duyff RF, Van den Bosch J, Laman DM, Potter van Loon BJ, Linssen WHJP. Neuromuscular findings in thyroid dysfunction: a prospective clinical and electrodiagnostic study. *J Neurol Neurosurg Psychiatry* 2000; **68**: 750–755.

Eslamian F, Bahrami A, Aghamohammadzadeh N, et al. Electrophysiologic changes in patients with primary hypothyroidism. *J Clin Neurophysiol* 2011; **28**: 323–328.

Klein I, Ojamaa K. Thyroid (neuro)myopathy. *Lancet* 2000; **356**: 614.

Video legends

The videos can be accessed at www.cambridge.org/9780521171854

Number	Title	Remarks
1.	Myotonic dystrophy type 1 (Case 50)	Action myotonia of hands (finger and wrist flexor muscles) and with hand grip Percussion myotonia of thenar muscles Steppage gait, more prominent with bare legs; walking on heels impossible Mild distal muscle atrophy of legs not arms Severe foot extensor muscle weakness
2.	Fasciculation in a healthy person	Sporadic fasciculation in posterior muscles of the legs (no voluntary muscle activity), no muscle atrophy
3.	Pyridostigmine-induced fasciculation of the tongue in a patient with classic myasthenia gravis	No atrophy of the tongue; fasciculation disappeared after reduction of the pyridostigmine dosage
4.	ALS (Case 1)	Atrophy of intrinsic hand and thenar muscles, and of biceps brachii with coarse fasciculation Hyperactive reflex of atrophic muscle Babinski and Chaddock reflexes with triple response of the leg
5.	Morvan's syndrome (Case 18)	Myokymia and fasciculation in muscles of leg, abdominal wall, and arm
6.	Pseudobulbar syndrome (Case 3)	Slow regular movements of an otherwise normal tongue (two patients) Concomitant movements of the jaw Hyperactive masseter reflex
7.	Becker muscular dystrophy (Case 38)	Gowers' sign; hyperlordosis Broad-based waddling gait (Duchenne gait)
8.	Miller–Fisher syndrome (Case 15)	Total ophthalmoplegia No facial weakness Mild arm weakness Sensory ataxia with finger–nose test Areflexia Ataxic gait
9.	Axial myopathy	Weak neck flexor muscles; no deltoid muscle weakness Weak erector trunci muscles Hyperlordosis obvious when walking
10.a	Kennedy disease (Case 5)	Limb girdle walking pattern Perioral and tongue fasciculation Postural and kinetic tremor Weakness of hip and knee flexor muscles
10.b	Kennedy disease (Case 5)	Weakness at closing of the eyes and when pouting and showing teeth Perioral and tongue fasciculation in a 53-year old man with Kennedy disease
11.	Distal myopathy (MMD3, see Table 44.1)	Examination of calves: no weak plantar flexion of the feet with legs extended (gastrocnemius muscles), weakness when walking (knees flexed: soleus muscles)
12.	Spastic gait in cervical stenosis with myelopathy lesion on MRI (Case 3)	Spastic ataxic gait more obvious when walking slowly in the consultation room compared with faster walking in the corridor. Note circumduction of the legs and side steps when turning Normal movements of the arms

Number	Title	Remarks
13.	Miller–Fisher syndrome (Case 15)	Completely bedridden patient Complete internal and external ophthalmoplegia with ptosis; no response to light Severe ataxia of the limbs
14.	Morvan's syndrome/neuromyotonia (Case 18)	First video before treatment: undulating myokymia, no weakness, profuse sweating Second video after treatment: decrease of myokymia, no sweating
15.	Neuropathy and ataxia caused by IgM-gammopathy (Case 20)	Mild postural and kinetic tremor Rombergism Ataxic broad-based gait
16.	Classic myasthenia gravis with ptosis (Case 34)	Provocation of asymmetric ptosis of the right eyelid when looking upwards, covering the pupil
17.	Becker muscular dystrophy (Case 38)	Gowers' sign Note hypertrophy of the calves
18.	Caveolinopathy-rippling muscle disease, including limb girdle muscular dystrophy (LGMD) type 1C (Case 39)	Pinching of the quadriceps femoris muscle causes rippling and mounding
19.	Calpainopathy-LGMD 2A (Case 40)	Waddling gait, hyperlordosis
20.	Calpainopathy-LGMD 2A (Case 40)	Gower's sign Atrophy of sternocostal part of pectoralis major muscles
21.	GSD II–Pompe disease (Case 53)	Mild weakness of abdominal wall muscles When walking, patient bends backward to remain stable

Index